CW00492522

"The APE Coach" Presents:

# IIFYM
# Flexible Dieting
# Bodybuilding Guide:

If It Fits Your Macros Diet Plan Trains You on How to Lose Weight, Build Muscle, Lose Body Fat, & Maintain a Healthy Lifestyle For the Perfect Physique!

TYLER JOHNSTON

www.APEcoach.com Presents:

# DISCLAIMER

First off, thank you for purchasing The "**IIFYM Flexible Dieting Bodybuilding Guide**" book. I hope you will enjoy everything you will find in it.

Every product I create, I pride myself on providing my customers, you, the very best information available in order to help you gain muscle, lose body fat, and achieve your ultimate fitness goals. To look your best, do your best and BE your best.

In exchange for this commitment, I would like you to make another one to me: do not copy, resell or steal this book without official permission.

You know just as well as I do that e-books are easily copied, shared and passed around. But you should know people like myself or other e-book writers make our living this way. I worked very hard for this book and am charging a very fair price for it, a price that you've also paid for this book. Therefore, if you know someone who'd like a copy, please send him or her my way.

This book is copyright, with all rights reserved. That means that all violations of this copyright (illegal copy, illegal distribution, illegal derivative works) are subject to legal action. In other words, don't make things messy for all of us by doing something illegal... My partners and affiliates actively search and often find all violations to my copyright.

Thanks for keeping your promises so I can continue doing my work and helping you with your fitness goals.

Thank you,

Tyler Johnston,
PTS, FNC, Amazon International Best-selling Author of "IIFYM Flexible Dieting Bodybuilding Guide".

P.S. The information in this book is for educational purposes only. It is not medical advice and is not intended to replace the advice or attention of health-care professionals. Consult your physician before beginning or making any changes in your diet or exercise program. Specific medical advice should be obtained from a licensed health-care practitioner.

Tyler Johnston and his associates will not assume any liability, nor be held responsible for any injury, illness or personal loss due to the utilization of any information contained herein.

Copyright © 2015 Tyler Johnston
All rights reserved.

# SPECIAL THANKS TO

I would like to send a special thanks to my mother Terra, father Ron, brother Rob, my girlfriend Tabitha, my friend and coach Scott, and my friend and mentor Luis.

Learn more about the amazing impact these individuals and many others have made in my life and fitness journey in the "Thank You Section".

# YOUR GIFTS

Get the "**IIFYM Flexible Dieting Bodybuilding Guide**" printable **Success Workbook** to set yourself up for greater success in your health, fitness and every area of your life.

Download Here:
**www.IIFYMBook.com/Extras**

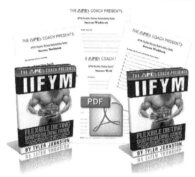

As a bonus, you will also get the **Ultimate Grocery List** with 50 of the most nutrient dense foods on the planet and their macros, a **Macro Cheat Sheet** to quickly and easily be able to determine the macronutrients in a huge variety of foods, and printable PDFs of the top **IIFYM Flexible Dieting Recipes** to include in your diet!

Get Access Now At:
**www.IIFYMBook.com/Extras**

# TESTIMONIALS

**What Others Say About Training with "The APE Coach" Tyler Johnston, IIFYM Flexible Dieting and Nutrition Coaching**

*– Jordan D, 23, Kitchener, CA*

"If you want a coach that really cares about you and your goals there is no one better for the job then Tyler… he sets you up to be able to live a healthy lifestyle and teaches you how to do it on your own… **In short if you're looking to get fit, shred pounds or get that dream body for the summer months at a good price and do it with someone you can call your friend, Tyler is the person you need to train with!**"

*– Alex C, 21, Kitchener, CA*

"Tyler is an amazing personal trainer! He personalizes your workouts and gives instructional videos to make working out easier…Tyler is **approachable with any issues you have about your health or any issues with workouts or meal plans.** I have allergies to certain foods and Tyler was able to cater to my problems."

*– Kevin A, 28, Baden, CA*

"I had hoped I could keep up with this and not fall off track again and Tyler has helped me do that… All of the positive feedback and support has been huge with keeping me on track. And the training plan has kept me focused especially with the help of the videos. I feel more confident… So far with training I have lost approximately 10lbs, have better understanding of healthy eating, gained confidence in my ability to start something and stick to it… **Overall this has been an amazing experience and I would recommend Tyler as a trainer and this program to anyone who asks!**"

*– Alley N, 22, Guelph, CA*

"With the nutrition guide, information on macro tracking and macro updates I've been able to achieve some great results! So far I have already gained strength and become more powerful, I can see my body becoming tighter/more toned, **I've lost 6lbs of fat and become much more knowledgeable on fuelling my body with the right macros!**"

*– Nicholas M, 19, Florida, USA*

"Before we started working together, I was a little hesitant on spending the money. I didn't have a job at the time and I know that health is a number one priority for me, but I wasn't sure if I was going to be able to pay for this program…
the cost turned out to be very reasonable and I made it happen! I have seen my body totally transform, my back looks amazing, now have a well-rounded knowledge about health and fitness, am more knowledgeable about exercise and nutrition, my strength has ridiculously improved! **Exercise is now a lifestyle for me and I am seeing results in my body every week. Tyler is awesome!**"

*– Matt, Amazon Kindle Reader, CA*

"Great read for anyone looking to make changes to their physique. Dieting is tough, but once you understand these concepts it can really help you take it to the next level. **I recommend this book to anyone and everyone!**"

*– Andrew, Amazon Kindle Reader, CA*

"A logical, practical approach to fitness and nutrition that sets you up for success. **I highly recommend this book!**"

# ABOUT THE AUTHOR

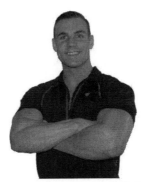

*Tyler Johnston "The APE Coach"*

- **Founder** and Head Training/ Fitness Nutrition Coach at Alpha Physique Engineering
- **Certified** Personal Training Specialist
- **Certified** Fitness Nutrition Coach
- **Won 1st** Men's Physique Medium at Guelph Mo-Muscle Classic
- **Won 1st** Mr. CHIN Fitness Model 2014
- **Nationally Qualified** CBBF Natural Men's Physique Competitor
- **Holds Degrees** in Psychology and Business Administration from Wilfrid Laurier University
- **Amazon International Best-selling Author** and Creator of "The APE Coach Presents" Series: IIFYM Flexible Dieting Bodybuilding Guide.

# LEARN MORE / CONTACT

Learn more about Tyler Johnston's "The APE Coach Presents" programs and other fitness and nutrition material for Bodybuilders, Physique Athletes, Fitness Beginners, Professionals, and everyone else, by going to: **www.APEcoach.com**

### SOCIAL
**FB:** www.Facebook.com/theAPEcoach
**YT:** www.Youtube.com/APEcoach
**IG:** @THEAPECOACH
**Twitter:** @THEAPECOACH
**Email:** info@APEcoach.com

# CONTENTS

www.APEcoach.com Presents:

# INTRODUCTION

Hi, I'm Tyler "The APE Coach", Personal Trainer, Fitness Nutrition Coach, Natural Physique Competitor, and Author. I want to start off by saying thank you and congratulations! By purchasing this book you are taking the first step towards building the body of your dreams and creating a healthier, happier lifestyle for the rest of your life!

I am so thrilled to have you join me here because the information in this book is everything I wish I knew when I first started my fitness journey. This approach to nutrition completely changed my life and allowed me to accomplish results in my physique that I never thought possible, and I know it will do the same for you!

I have to say, I feel you and I must be kindred spirits because this is exactly how I started out in my personal fitness journey. I was hungry for information and knew there had to be something out there, some better information that truly produced results. So I searched through blogs and forums and books and read tons of e-books just like this one! I really attribute a lot of the success I've been able to accomplish in my health and fitness to that relentless search for knowledge and the reading I was fortunate enough to come across early on.

And so, by having you here with me I am so excited for you, because you are one of the few who doesn't settle for average, you are an achiever. You look for ways to constantly improve, to better yourself and to be outstanding!

As I mentioned, this book contains all the information on nutrition that I wish I had when I first started. Growing up, I was always very active as a kid playing multiple sports all throughout the year, hockey, soccer, baseball, etc. I had a pretty solid foundation when it came to fitness and exercise but where I always struggled was nutrition.

With so much, seemingly contradictory, information out in the media and magazines on what a healthy diet and nutrition plan is, I was lost. But I was determined to not let that stop me; when I began working out I worked my ass off and trained as hard as I could every single time I grabbed a weight. Because of this, I was fortunate enough to get some pretty great results. From the time I started weightlifting in grade 11 until the summer after high school, I was able to put on about 15-20lbs of muscle.

I was extremely happy and proud of myself, but I knew there had to be more. I tried to stick to one of the chicken, broccoli and tuna bodybuilding diets multiple times but I just couldn't keep to it long-term. I would stick to it for about a month, think I was doing great but not really see any significant differences and would eventually go back to Mini Pizzas, KD, and Reese Puffs. And surprisingly, the results weren't all that different… Something wasn't adding up.

I read article after article and post after post about how nutrition is so important for building muscle and burning fat yet I wasn't seeing very big differences from when I was eating "clean" to when I was eating "junk". Originally, the whole genetics argument crept in to my head and that's what people would tell me; oh you must just have good genes, it's just your genes, your biochemistry.

But I don't buy that; yes it may play a role and be one factor, but if it was entirely our genes, than anyone overweight with high body fat would never become skinny and muscular; anyone skinny would never become obese, yet I've seen hundreds of examples of each. Moreover, if you've ever heard any of Tony Robbins' seminars or other personal development speakers and success coaches, you'll know we can change our biochemistry in a heartbeat simply by what we feel and what we focus on.

So I wouldn't accept genes as the answer. I knew there had to be some reason that I was still able to put on muscle and maintain relatively low body fat while not eating very "clean" at all. Mind you, I always ate a lot of chicken and meat and always ensured I got lots and lots of protein… even with the mini pizzas and grilled cheese.

I was stumped; after reading over and over, it is impossible to build muscle or burn fat without eating "clean", how could I? I wasn't getting the results I really dreamed of, but I was getting results. So I searched and searched, how could it be that I could still get any results eating junk? Was nutrition not as important as everyone said it was? Could you just get results from busting your ass in the gym hard enough? Or were the types of foods not as important?

Finally I came across Flexible Dieting. Suddenly, it all made sense...

I realized that I was in a sense following the principles of Flexible Dieting without realizing it or really measuring my results. Because of this, I could still get decent results and put on some muscle mass even while eating junk. It wasn't until I understood Flexible Dieting in its entirety though, that I was able to manifest the incredible results I've achieved now.

Once I discovered the true power of Flexible Dieting, my strength, size and overall physique completely transformed to a level I never even imagined possible for myself before. I was able to eat quite literally anything I wanted, within moderation, and step on stage with a natural physique that took home first place trophies!

After the incredible results I was able to achieve with this unique approach to nutrition myself, and discovering how thousands of other fitness competitors and bodybuilders used the same principles for nutrition, I was hooked. I finally understood how these magazine cover fitness models were able to keep such amazing physiques all year round without going insane from "eating clean".

I was ecstatic with my discovery, and yet at the same time I was a little outraged. Why wasn't this information fully available to everyone?! Why wasn't this amazing approach to nutrition that would solve so many dietary problems we see these days common knowledge to everyone?! Why was it being kept to just the "in-crowd" in the fitness industry?

I knew I had to make a change! I had to get this life-changing information out to as many individuals as I possibly could! Too many people are suffering from nutritional related health issues and diseases. Too many people are suffering from a complete lack of self-confidence and self-respect due to their physical appearance. But no more! It is my mission to share this vital knowledge with as many individuals on this planet that I possibly can.

I now work in the fitness industry because it is my utmost passion in life. Not only do I live and breathe fitness and health in my day to day life now, I specialize in helping others achieve results in their fitness and health. I am so grateful now to be able to work with individuals all across the world achieve real results and transformations in their fitness, health, nutrition, and physiques! From teens looking to pack on lean muscle mass, to middle-aged folks wanting to get back into the best shape of their lives, those who have never exercised or dieted before, to those stepping on stage at a fitness show. I have had the pleasure to work with people from numerous backgrounds each with different goals.

With Online Personal Training, Fitness and Nutrition Coaching, my clients and I work together to come up with a plan that is specific to their individual needs, goals and lifestyles to ensure their ultimate success. Additionally, I ensure my clients are motivated, inspired and educated to allow them to maintain their incredible results long after our time working together has ended.

I don't believe in hiding information or setting clients up to be dependent on their trainer for results. I believe in offering the very best of my abilities and providing the greatest service I possibly can to ensure my clients achieve their ultimate dreams and goals with their health and fitness. And I believe in educating and empowering each of my clients to be able to adhere to the healthy lifestyle changes in the future to maintain their dream physiques!

The principles discussed in this book are the key that have allowed my clients and me to achieve such incredible results and now I am honoured to share them with you.

This is the guide that will train you to finally create the body of your dreams eating foods you love!

No more nonsense restrictive, "magic food" diets portrayed in the media. No more starving yourself and eating bland flavourless food that makes you miserable. No more 1000 Calorie or less crash diets that allow you to lose 10lbs in a week only to gain 15lbs the following week when you can no longer stick to the ridiculous rules. It's time to stop the BS pushed out in the media and show you the truth! It's time you became part of the "in-crowd". It's time for you to truly create the body of your dreams!

Now, if you're wondering if this only works for athletes or bodybuilders or those with extensive knowledge in exercise and nutrition, have no fear! This book is designed to train you how to understand nutrition at a whole new level and step you through the process one step at a time. The most effective way to achieve great results is through taking action, and the best way to ensure individuals are able to take action is to make it as simple as possible. This book is designed to take you through the simple steps that set you up for action! And to achieve your ultimate fitness and health goals and anyone can do it!

Take my own, lovely mother for example. She has never studied exercise or nutrition nor has she read literature regarding proper exercise or nutrition principles, other than the occasional pop-culture magazine. I had her sit down one night to help proof-read through this book and hear what she thought of it. She read through, found a couple typos and offered some suggestions, which was great!

Then she asked me, "So this is all I have to do to lose weight?"

"Yes. It's easy".

"And I can still eat a sub or pizza and have a cookie at lunch?"

"Yes. You don't have to cut out any of the regular foods from your diet. That's the beauty of flexible dieting!"

So she decided to give it a shot, she followed the simple steps at the end of this book to get started and adhered to the principles laid out in this book to see if it would work. A couple weeks later, she noticed her pants fitting looser and told me how she had been losing a lot of weight from following the book. Fast forward to about 12 weeks now, and she's lost over 20lbs and ALL of her clothes are loose on her!

Looks like it's time for a shopping spree.

It has been so great hearing how happy she has been over the past few weeks updating me on all the weight she has lost. And I can really see that she feels so much better achieving her goals without having to restrict herself to a limit of foods. She was joking with me and said how she's been able to lose all this weight and she can still eat pizza for lunch every day! But the funny thing is, she can and she does! She makes homemade flatbread pizzas that fit her macros and the results keep coming!

I am so happy to have been able to help her achieve such amazing results with this book and show her that losing weight and looking great doesn't have to be so difficult. That is the beauty of this, it can be fun, enjoyable and exciting to get in the best shape of your life, and it should be! I know if she was able to get such great results with no prior knowledge of fitness and nutrition just by following the simple steps in this book, you absolutely can too!

Let this book be your personal guide, your introduction into a whole new world of understanding nutrition. You will finally be able to create the body of your dreams eating foods you love AND be able to enjoy the process!

Welcome to… The APE Coach Presents: IIFYM Flexible Dieting Bodybuilding Guide!

## *Chapter I*
# FLEXIBLE DIETING?

### What The Heck is IIFYM?

I know what you're thinking... get the body of my dreams eating foods I love? I love cheesecake, burgers and ice cream; are you telling me I can get the body of my dreams eating this?

My answer to this is simply, well... yes. Within moderation you can eat ALL these foods while still achieving your fitness goals and look great.

How is that possible you ask? I thought you have to eat "clean" and eliminate all junk and sugar and fat and carbs. Now you're telling me the complete opposite of that!

Introducing... Flexible Dieting! Or as it's commonly referred to, If It Fits Your Macros (IIFYM).

Flexible dieting is a new approach to eating that runs contrary to traditional dietary approaches. This is important because a lot of traditional approaches seem to fail. Let's take a look at why this is the case.

### Why Traditional Dieting Fails:

Lyle McDonald, in his book *A Guide to Flexible Dieting*, lays out what he believes are the 2 main reasons traditional dieting fails

1) Being too absolute and expecting perfection.
2) Focusing only on the short-term.

We know it all too well, you find yourself overweight, out of shape and you want to be lean and strong yesterday.

So you drastically cut calories, start eating like a rabbit filling your plates with veggies and salads choking down your bite-sized dishes and exercising like crazy. Within a short period of time you're losing weight and tell yourself; this tastes awful but it is working great, and you deal with being miserable because you know it will pay off. And it does work… for the short-term, but it won't long term.

Eventually you find it too difficult to maintain your diet while maintaining your sanity and you begin to slip, giving into temptations and cravings. Finally you hit the wall and binge like a mad man who's been famished for 4 weeks and just let into King's Buffet free of charge! Ultimately you lose all your hard earned progress and then some, setting yourself back even further on your lean body journey.

The guilt piles on, you feel like a complete failure and you come to the conclusion that you just are the way you are. You tried to lose weight and have enough willpower to stick to your diet, but you just couldn't do it any longer.

A good friend of mine, and now client, certainly had some experience with this, one too many times. He came to me in distress about his health and fitness. He had hit a record high in his body weight at 210lbs and decided it was time to get some help and take care of this once and for all.

He explained to me how the past few years he had attempted to lose weight and get in shape several times before and he would really be motivated and set on achieving his goals. He had the best intentions to achieve results and work as hard as he needed to really make it happen. However, every year something would come up and inevitably, he would end up falling off track and reverting back to where he was beforehand or worse.

It was a constant cycle of overweight, time to get in shape, start to lose weight, fall off, gain it back and repeat. No matter how hard he worked or how motivated he was at the start, he just couldn't maintain his results and it started to seem like nothing was going to work. Sound familiar to any of you?

Well, I've got news for you, you were set up! That's right, that super strict diet and drastic lifestyle change was setting you up for failure from the start! And you're not alone; too many people are set up to fail just the same and we're going to stop it here and now.

The truth is that you'll lose more fat, faster, and easier by giving yourself a break here and there. Flexible dieting is really the opposite of this traditional restrictive and rigid approach.

Instead of forcing yourself to follow strict unsustainable rules to lose weight and be healthy, you take a more relaxed, long-term perspective with your diet. In this book, you'll learn the general principles of "flexible dieting", to be less strict about your diet and get amazing results, without going insane. That's the essence of flexible dieting. Keep it Simple!

So to get back to my good friend, we started working together and I had him apply all of the concepts in this book for his nutrition and set him up on a solid training plan that suits his needs and his busy lifestyle.

The results? He's been able to achieve a steady, healthy pace of weight loss, losing about 1lb each week and his strength has sky rocketed! Even with a random bout of Shingles, and complications that would have normally thrown his results completely out the window and knocked him off track entirely, he was able to stay the course! We simply had 1 week of a minor setback, adjusted for it and got right back on track with no issues!

The flexible dieting principles from this book are what really saved him and allowed him to stay on track with his goals even with an unexpected set back.

So if you've ever found yourself in a similar situation or not known how to stick to your plan whenever setbacks would arise (believe me, somehow they always arise), then you're in luck!

This book will explain exactly how you can easily work around setbacks and continue right on track. No more cycles, no more unreasonable guilt, no more set-ups for failure. If you follow the information in this book, you will succeed!

## *Chapter II*
# HOW FLEXIBLE DIETING WORKS

**Macros vs. Calories:**

Flexible Dieting (IIFYM) is simply the tracking of macronutrients (Protein, Carbohydrates, Fats) to attain a desired body composition goal.

Macronutrients make up the bulk of our diet and each has a caloric value:

| | |
|---|---|
| *1 gram protein* | *= 4 calories* |
| *1 gram carbohydrate* | *= 4 calories* |
| *1 gram fat* | *= 9 calories* |

Instead of the typical calorie counting approach (i.e. Eating 2500 Calories a day), flexible dieters track macronutrients instead (i.e. 225g Protein, 276g Carbohydrate, 55g Fat = 2500 Calories).

In Chapters 10 through 16 of this book you will learn exactly how to do this quickly and easily. So don't worry if this seems a little confusing to you at first.

**Weight Loss and Weight Gain: Understanding Calories**

Weight gain and weight loss generally comes down to a calorie surplus (Eating more calories than you burn in a day) or calorie deficit (Eating less calories than you burn in a day) respectively. Although the '*type*' of weight lost or gained is directly influenced by the ratio of macronutrients you consume day to day.

It has been typically stated in research that 1lb of bodyweight equals about 3500 Calories. This means if you are wanting to lose 1lb of bodyweight in one week, you need to consume approximately 500 Calories less than you burn each day (500 Calories x 7 days = 3500 Calories / week).

To illustrate this further, see the diagram on the next page: **Calories** affect **weight loss** or **weight gain**. (Lighter vs. Heavier)

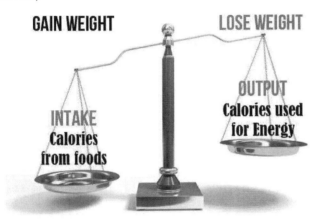

**Calorie Surplus** – More Calories in + Less Calories Out = Weight Gain

**Calorie Deficit** – Less Calories in + More Calories Out = Weight Loss

## Changing Body Composition: Understanding Macros

**Macronutrients** affect **body composition** (Muscle mass vs. Fat mass)

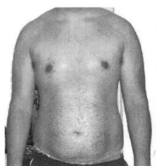 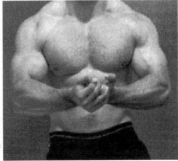

Both guys are 190 lbs...

**Proper Macronutrients** = Lean Muscle Mass + Power

**Improper Macronutrients** = High Body Fat % + Weakness

As you can see, there is a lot more to it than simply calories in vs. calories out when it comes to body composition. If you want to be 190lbs of solid muscle rather than 190lbs of soft flab, the *type* of calories you eat (*macronutrients*) is what's really important.

**A Calorie is a Calorie, A Macro is a Macro:**
So that means I've gotta eat "clean" now, right? Nope!

At least, not entirely, Flexible Dieting follows an understanding that there are no "clean" or "dirty" foods, no "miracle weight loss foods", no be-all, end-all magic diet that is better than all the rest. To repeat, this means there are no good or bad foods, just macronutrient ratios.

The body does not discern between 10g of carbohydrate from maple syrup for example (a "dirty" food), and 10g of carbohydrates from sweet potato (a "clean" food). 10 grams of carbohydrates = 10 grams of carbohydrates no matter what the source, period.

Let's further illustrate this point, shall we?

Here, we have:

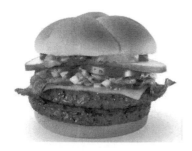

**A Bacon Double Cheeseburger:**
- **34g Protein**
- **39g Carbohydrate**
- **39g Fat**

OR

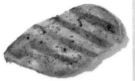 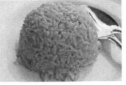 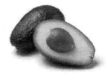

**A Chicken Breast, Brown Rice and an Avocado:**
- **34g Protein**
- **39g Carbohydrate**
- **39g Fat**

Both have the same macronutrient values, therefore both will achieve the same results in your body composition. It is simple science.

Your body does not think to itself "is this healthy or unhealthy"?

When food enters the stomach; it simply breaks down the food and processes the macronutrients.

A calorie is a calorie, and a macro is a macro; this is further emphasized in the *"Twinkie Diet"* where Dr. Mark Haub ate nothing but Twinkies and a couple other sugary snack foods, 3 times a day for 10 weeks instead of meals and was able to lose 27 pounds.

Now this is simply to illustrate that calories are what ultimately impact weight loss or weight gain, but to re-iterate if you are wanting to lose *fat* and gain *muscle* your macronutrients are what make the difference in your overall body composition or what type of weight is lost or gained.

Now before you go off on a bulk barn binge or a full-out assault on me. There are some differences in food sources that can be more or less nutritious for you.

Foods also contain important micronutrients and phytonutrients such as vitamins, minerals and fiber (many consider fiber to be a

4th macro nutrient because it is so important for proper digestive health and regularity in the body). These micronutrients, phytonutrients and fiber are extremely important in overall health and well-being because if you are deficient in any of these vitamins or minerals, it can dramatically impact your levels of performance and energy, and can quickly put a halt to fat loss and muscle building efforts.

Due to the high impact and importance of these additional nutrients in your diet, high emphasis should be placed on ensuring you are getting quality food sources such as lean proteins and vegetables. These foods contain these essential nutrients and fiber (as a general guideline Males typically should consume 38g of Fiber per day and Females 25g Fiber per day according to the Institute of Medicine).

This does not mean however, that 100% of your diet has to be lean chicken breast and broccoli! For a general rule of thumb to get exceptional results in improving your body composition and really creating that body of your dreams you can follow the 80/20 rule.

To clarify, if you make sure to get 80% of your daily foods from quality nutritious food sources including your lean proteins and lots of vegetables, the last 20% can come from foods of your choice!

So if you feel like having a brownie with some ice cream, not a problem! As long as the majority of your diet is coming from more nutrient dense foods you can still work in all of your favourite foods to your daily diet without sacrificing your results! This is the beauty of flexible dieting!

**What about the Mysterious Metabolism?**

Now I did my best to step through how calories affect the body and weight loss and then how macronutrients affect the body. But I know you've heard this word a thousand times "*metabolism*" and some of you may be wondering how that plays a role in this process.

So what is your *metabolism*?

Essentially, metabolism is a sum of chemical processes in the cells of your body where some substances are broken down to create energy for vital functions and activities within the body and other substances are assimilated by the body to maintain life.

How does this relate to fitness or weight loss? Well calories that we consume are broken down by the metabolism to provide our bodies with energy. If we consume more calories than the metabolism can "burn" for energy, the excess is stored in our body. This is essentially how we accumulate fat in the body. If you remember from the previous section on calories, this would be what is considered a "caloric surplus". So I'm sure you can imagine how a deficit is created as well.

Some people have a "faster metabolism" meaning their bodies naturally burn more calories for energy and thus they can consume more calories than others of the same weight without gaining weight. Some have "slower metabolisms" meaning their bodies naturally burn less calories for energy and store more of it on their body. This is why everyone knows that one person who can eat anything they want and never seems to gain a pound. Vice versa for some it seems like no matter what they eat they seem to gain weight or at least never lose weight. Like everything in life, each individual has a different metabolism.

Now I don't want to get too in depth with metabolism because that is not the focus of this book. But I do want to ensure you understand what it is and how it plays a role with your fitness goals because it is a crucial component. I also want you to understand that it is not static. Meaning it is not simply set at one specific point. Your metabolism changes and adapts to the amount of energy you supply your body (i.e. the amount of calories you consume) and the type of energy you supply it (i.e. the macros you consume).

When you are in a caloric surplus, your metabolism speeds up to try to burn more of this energy, when you are in a caloric deficit, your metabolism slows down because there is not as much energy needed to burn. This means when you are eating more your metabolism works harder to burn more and makes it harder to put on weight. And when you are eating less (i.e. dieting) your metabolism slows down making it harder to lose weight. This is why some seem to struggle like hell to gain a pound and others struggle like hell to lose one.

## Why Does It Speed Up and Slow Down?

Naturally, your metabolism likes to keep your bodyweight within a certain range, sort of like a thermostat. If you've got the temperature set at 70° and the room drops to 62°, the heater kicks on and it heats back up to 70°. Likewise if it gets too hot the air conditioning kicks on and cools it down. Your metabolism works in a very similar way.

If you provide your body with more and more energy (calories), your metabolism goes "woah, this is getting to be too much" and the metabolism speeds up and burns more energy to try to keep your weight where it is at within its' comfortable range. Similarly if you go on a super restrictive diet, providing your body with an almond wrapped in a spinach leaf, your metabolism again goes "wtf?! I'm not getting anything from outside, so whatever comes in I am not burning; I am storing this as fat as long as I can so that I don't die." The metabolism slows to try to keep you up at the same weight you were at.

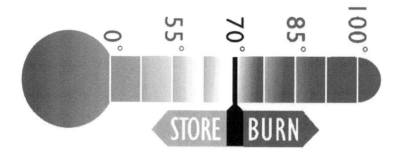

This is why if you try to rush things and go to extremes, you often fail and quick. There is a reason crash diets are called crash diets. Because you provide your body with so little energy, such a small amount of food that your metabolism literally crashes to a halt. If you cut out too much too quick your metabolism drops right down to keep you at the weight you were at and then makes it nearly impossible to continue losing weight.

This is how a metabolism gets "damaged" and it can be very, very hard to "repair" and build back up after the damage is done. So please, the next time you see some super restrictive under 1000 calorie supermodel diet, for the love of everything holy, don't do it! More extreme does not equal better results in the world of health and nutrition!

Now, although your metabolism typically stays at a certain point, unlike popular belief, this is not a single rigid, set point that can never be changed.

I alluded already to the ability to "repair" and "build up" a damaged metabolism; yes it is possible to change the speed of your metabolism or how efficiently it burns energy.

I know, from first-hand experience, from working with many clients, discussing with colleagues and reading studies that your metabolism can be adjusted over time to some extent. So instead of thinking of your metabolism being set in stone at a certain level, a better way to think of it is a settling point or a temporary rest stop.

When you consistently provide your body a certain amount of energy (calories) your metabolism gets used to that amount so to speak. So if you make slow, gradual changes and allow the body and metabolism to progress and adjust, you can speed up or slow down the metabolism over time this way. But again, this takes very specific individual attention and is beyond the scope of this book.

So if you would like to know more about this and would like help from yours truly, "*The APE Coach*", to really get the most out of your training and nutrition, you can apply to my exclusive online coaching program at (www.APEcoach.com/Coaching) for a complete individualized plan and ongoing coaching and program adjustments directly from me.

*Please note, due to high demand and my focus on providing the best possible service to each and every client I work with, not everyone may be accepted for the program. But I'd love to hear from you and I will be in touch with you regardless.*

**The Metabolism Engine:**

So we've just gone through a ton of information. We've covered calories, macros and metabolism, in a fair amount of detail. But I want to make sure everyone fully understands this section because it is crucial for achieving your fitness and health goals.

In order to help further explain how your metabolism, calories, macronutrients, weight loss and body composition are all related, I came up with a metaphor. I find this the easiest way to explain how your metabolism works and why calories aren't the only factor for weight loss or changes in body composition. So let's jump right into it!

I call this the metabolism engine, and it works like this:
1. Your body's metabolism is like an engine.
2. The calories you put into your body is like engine oil.
3. The macros that make up those calories are the quality of oil you put in.

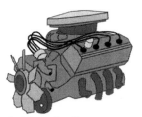 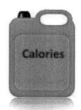 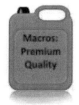

**1. Metabolism          2. Calories          3. Macros**

Your metabolism needs energy (calories) to run, much like an engine needs oil to run.

And much like an engine in a car, the amount of oil has to be within a certain range (between the min and max fill lines) in order for the engine to operate the most efficiently. This is the same with your metabolism and calories. The calorie intake has to be within the metabolism's comfortable range for it to run the most efficiently. Too little calories, the metabolism slows as the "engine" doesn't have enough "oil" to keep things running full speed. Too many calories, the metabolism starts burning the excess like crazy, the "engine" starts burning all the excess "oil".

Finally, the quality of oil that you put in your engine effects how well it is able to perform. If you put dirty, old sludgy oil in your engine, it's not going to run well. But if you put top of the line premium oil designed for that specific engine, it hums along running at full performance smooth as can be. So the macros (oil type), or quality of the calories (oil) you put in, dramatically affect how well the metabolism (engine) is able to perform and function.

So you need to be sure, whenever making changes to your diet or nutrition, they are made properly and gradually. Patience is quite a virtue when it comes to improving your metabolism and changing your body composition.

Slow and steady progress is better than a 10 second mile into the wall!

*Chapter III*
# BONUS –
# THE ULTIMATE GROCERY LIST

### 10 of the Top Nutritious and Nutrient Dense Foods:

Now that we've covered all the basics, I want to help get you started at understanding foods and macros. I've included a list here of 10 of the most nutritious and nutrient dense foods that would be great to include in your diet, along with the macros for each. This will help you determine what foods are more nutritious or "nutrient dense" and what sort of macros different foods have.

1.  **Eggs** – among the most nutritious foods on the planet. Most bioavailable source of protein and loaded with healthy fats. **Macros Per 1 Large Egg – 73 Calories | 6g Protein | 0.5g Carbs | 5g Fat**

2.  **Avocado** – Different than most other fruits, avocado is loaded with healthy fats instead of carbs. They are high in fiber, potassium and Vitamin C **Macros Per 1 Avocado – 322 Calories | 4g Protein | 17g Carbs | 29.5g Fat**

3.  **Chicken Breast** – Extremely high in protein and low in fat and calories. **Macros Per 3oz Chicken Breast – 135 Calories | 27g Protein | 0g Carbs | 3g Fat**

4.  **Chia Seeds** – Among the most nutrient dense foods on the planet. Very high in fiber, magnesium, manganese, calcium and various other nutrients. **Macros Per 15g Chia Seeds – 65 | 3g Protein | 6g Carbs | 5g Fat**

5.  **Broccoli** – An excellent source of fiber, vitamin K and vitamin C. Also contains a high amount of protein compared to most other vegetables.
    **Macros Per 100g Broccoli – 35 Calories | 2.4g Protein | 7.2g Carbs | 0.4g Fat**

6.  **Spinach** – Most of the calories in spinach come from protein. Spinach is one of the best sources of potassium, magnesium and provides iron, and plenty vitamins and minerals.
    **Macros Per 100g Spinach – 23 Calories | 2.9g Protein | 3.6g Carbs | 0.4g Fat**

7.  **Salmon** – Excellent source of protein and Omega-3 fatty acids. Also contains vitamin D and many other nutrients.
    **Macros Per 3oz Salmon – 155 Calories | 21.6g Protein | 0g Carbs | 6.9g Fat**

8.  **Oats** – Incredibly healthy, loaded with nutrients and contain powerful fibers called beta-glucans that help with digestive health.
    **Macros Per 90g Oats – 330 Calories | 15g Protein | 60g Carbs | 6g Fat**

9.  **Sweet Potatoes** – Loaded with antioxidants and lots of healthy nutrients. Also one of the tastiest starchy foods you can eat.
    **Macros Per 3oz Sweet Potato – 75 Calories | 1.8g Protein | 17.4g Carbs | 0g Fat**

10. **Apples** – High in fiber and contain plenty of antioxidants and vitamin C
    **Macros Per 100g Apple – 52 Calories | 0.3g Protein | 13.8g Carbs | 0.2g Fat**

AND as an added BONUS and a THANK YOU for purchasing this book:

I've created "The Ultimate Grocery List for Losing Weight, Building Muscle, Burning Fat and Maintaining a Healthy Lifestyle: 50 of The Most Nutritious and Nutrient Dense Foods on The Planet!"

You can get your **FREE** copy of the complete list of the top 50 most nutritious and nutrient dense foods on the planet by visiting www.IIFYMbook.com/Ultimate-Grocery-List and downloading the list which also has each food's macronutrients!

*Chapter IV*

# THE PSYCHOLOGY OF EATING

### The Inner Game: It's Not All Physical!

Allowing yourself "cheat" foods in your diet in moderation doesn't have to completely derail your entire nutrition plan and destroy your fat loss or muscle building results. In fact, incorporating these foods can do wonders for your psychological state when following a nutrition plan or diet.

Most individuals and most media only focus on the physical aspect of dieting or changing your dietary and lifestyle habits, but nutrition and exercise is certainly not just physical. There is a large emotional and psychological response in the body that often gets ignored or down-played. Our thoughts and emotions about food play a major role when dieting and are crucial elements to achieving overall success.

For this reason, I have devoted an entire section of this book to the topic of the psychology of eating. In this section you will learn why we over-eat, what causes us to like or loath certain foods and how to take a healthier approach to dieting and nutrition.

### Emotional Eating and Why We Over-Eat:

Many individuals who are overweight find themselves eating much more than they should be without knowing why. Sometimes they don't even have conscious awareness of it, other times they feel they cannot control their over-eating. A large reason for this is that we, as humans are emotional beings. We do not simply operate on logic or statistics alone like robots, we have emotional responses to everything and food is no exception. The reason people over-eat is largely due to positive emotions people have linked up in their brain to certain foods.

The way we learn is through conditioning. We are constantly

being bombarded with different stimuli and over time our emotional states can become linked up with a specific stimulus in our brains. This sounds complicated, but it's really easy.

Let's clarify this with an example. Take coffee for instance. Coffee has a very distinct taste; the taste of coffee is the stimulus. Now the first time you tasted plain, black coffee, what was your response?

Did you say "Oh boy, this tastes fantastic; I can't wait to drink 3 of these a day!"

I doubt that very seriously.

So why then do so many people drink coffee every single day to the point of addiction?

Because after a few times drinking the coffee, (and maybe with some sweeteners and milk or cream), they got this rush of energy.

With all this extra energy they felt great, they were in this positive emotional state, and what happened was somewhere along the line, they began to link up in their brain coffee equals energy, feeling great and pleasure.

So eventually they became *conditioned* to feel positive *emotional responses* to the taste (or *stimulus*) of the coffee. This is the reason that people say coffee is an "acquired taste" because until you become *conditioned* to link positive emotions and feelings with the taste of coffee, you generally don't really like it.

This same thing is happening all the time with the foods we eat as well, and a lot of times we don't even realize it. This is why we can find ourselves feeling out of control with our eating, or find ourselves at the end of a movie having eaten an entire bag of chips when we weren't even hungry.

Our brain does whatever it can to avoid pain and to gain pleasure. So overtime we become conditioned with emotional responses to certain foods and our brain links up that a piece of chocolate cake for example, equals massive pleasure so we eat a lot of it. The same can be true with more nutritious foods. Maybe as a child having to eat a plate of brussel sprouts was a form of punishment, or you had some vegetables that you really didn't like, so you linked up that these vegetables and nutritious foods equal pain and you avoid them.

So by following a more flexible approach with your diet and sources of nutrition, it becomes much easier to adhere to your nutrition plan in the long run and really make lasting lifestyle changes. This is a much healthier approach to changing your eating habits rather than restricting yourself to a specific set of foods and going through pain until you can't take it anymore and your brain goes "I've had it! I can't stay on this diet any longer; I feel like I'm dying!"

**Maintaining Fat Loss: Just as Important as Achieving It**

If you are a rigid dieter it is likely you think in the short term with your diet for a couple reasons:

1. You want results as fast as possible, so you follow a restrictive diet you hate and rationalize that it's okay for now because it won't last long.

2. With the restrictive diet, you become even more focused on the short term because that's the only way you can bear to stay on it.

Sometimes you might actually reach your goal with this approach. But losing fat isn't really the hard part. Maintaining fat loss is.

This is where restrictive dieting approaches almost always fail. The behaviours that help you lose fat are the same ones that will help you stay lean, so if you can't maintain the exercise and nutrition habits that helped you lose fat, you probably won't be able to stay lean long term.

Studies have repeatedly shown that meal replacements and weight loss shakes help people lose a lot of weight. It helps them control their portion sizes and total caloric intake. The problem is that these people never learn how to control their calories and portions without the shakes and meal replacements. They don't learn how to maintain weight loss with sustainable enjoyable habits. That is why longer studies generally show that meal replacements are not very effective in helping people maintain much weight loss, if any at all.

The key to really creating that body of your dreams is consistent improvements and adherence to better lifestyle choices and behaviours in your fitness and nutrition. By allowing yourself to have foods you love in moderation it becomes a lot less painful and so much more rewarding in the long run as you see the dramatic improvements in your body composition and your health.

Flexible dieting can set you free from feeling utterly deprived and restricted on the typical "clean diet" and allows you to maintain a more healthy relationship with food on an emotional and psychological level. Being too restrictive or too extreme is a recipe for developing eating disorders, which can be very serious and very harmful to the body.

So give yourself a break and focus on the long-term outcome not the quick-fix. Let's reverse this misinformed trend. There is nothing wrong with loving the journey towards improving your health and your physique; a healthy lifestyle doesn't have to equal pain!

Instead of seeing your diet as a temporary obstacle to forget about once you've gotten lean, think of it as a long term transition to healthier habits and lifestyle changes that you'll use to stay lean for the rest of your life.

*Chapter V*

# SETTING UP FOR SUCCESS

Now before we jump in to the action steps and get you started on building that body of your dreams, I want to make sure you are absolutely 100% set up for success.

I don't want this to be just another diet book you read and put on the shelf. I want this to be unlike anything you've ever read on diet and nutrition before! I want this to be a book you can digest and immediately be able to put into action to produce dramatic improvements in the quality of your life.

I don't just want to give you a bunch of facts and information and leave you to make sense of it all like most other books do. I want to ensure you have every resource necessary to produce extraordinary results and completely transform your life for the better.

By applying the tools and principles in this book, you will be able to achieve excellence in any area of your life. This book is your blueprint to excellence and success, not only in your nutrition and health, but in your life as well.

Now in order to fully cover this topic, it really requires a complete book of its own. So if you would like to read into greater depth and detail on this topic, you can get my book on Ultimate Fitness Lifestyle Success at www.IIFYMbook.com/Success-Book.

My job and my desire is to help you achieve results! So in this section I want to cover some key steps to success and ensure you are completely set up and ready to achieve your goals whatever they may be. And the best thing about this, is that this can be applied to any area of your life that you want to achieve greater success in. Whether you want to improve your fitness and health, your relationships, your finances, your family life, or your career, this will allow you to achieve greater results than ever before.

So let's get right to it! How do we achieve anything we want in life and how can we set ourselves up to be totally successful?

What does it take to be successful? What separates the achievers from the failures?

The super successful from the merely average?

Why is it that some people seem to struggle in spite of every opportunity, while others thrive and succeed through the most difficult situations imaginable?

I believe the key to success and the one thing that separates the achievers from the non-achievers is their ability to take *consistent action*! Those that succeed on a major level have an uncanny ability to consistently get themselves to take action no matter what the circumstances.

Success is not an accident. It is not just by some random roll of a dice that some people succeed far beyond the rest of society. There are specific things that successful people do consistently to produce the quality of results that turn their dreams into their everyday reality. And if you pay attention, learn what they do, and how they do it, you can model this and create similar results in your own life. Now, I want to show you exactly how.

The actions that all achievers take make up a powerful formula for success.

## So What Is The Formula For Success?

I believe it can be broken down into 5 simple steps.

## 1) They Know Their Result!

They know exactly what they want their end-result to be. They have a crystal clear vision of exactly what they want to have, be, and do. They also know why they want it. They have a burning desire to accomplish their goal, almost an obsession that literally pulls them towards its attainment. This is the first crucial step to achieving anything you want. You have to have a clear vision and you must have a reason, with a burning desire that excites you and propels you towards your goals through any and all conditions.

## 2) They Take Action!

They formulate a strategy or blueprint that can get them from where they are now to where they want to be and they take consistent action towards their goal. They don't try to plan out every single detail and think of all the difficulties they will have to overcome to accomplish their dreams and become overwhelmed.

They simply lay out one possible strategy, determine what single action will take them one step closer to reaching their goal and they act on it. And they continue doing this consistently, one step, after another, after another. Additionally, they commit to doing whatever it takes to achieve their result, no matter what the consequences, no matter what others say or think, no matter how realistic or unrealistic it may seem. They absolutely refuse to give up on their goal, and will keep trying relentlessly, unwavering, until they accomplish their vision or die trying.

## 3) They Have Result Oriented Awareness (ROA).

All this means is they are simply aware of the results they are producing and in what direction it is taking them. Every time they take an action step and produce a result, they are evaluating to be aware, is this taking me closer to my result or further away? This leads them to the fourth step of success, which is:

## 4) They Change Their Approach

If they know their result, they take action, and they discover they are not heading towards their goal; or they try something and fail. They simply change their approach, determine a new action that can take them one step closer to their vision and continue on their path to success. The road to success is very rarely a clear straight laneway, there are many twists and turns to maneuver and many bumps and obstacles to overcome. Whenever they realize they are off course from their ultimate end-result, they change their approach to bring them back on track. They understand that this is a continual process, it takes constant revision and updating to keep progressing towards the end-result. Finally, they take step five, which is:

## 5) They See Past Themselves.

The most successful individuals always find a way to give something back. To contribute to others beyond themselves in need of their help. The way the super successful really achieve excellence in the quality of their life is by providing value to others and improving others' lives as well as their own. This contribution to society is what really takes their life from good or great and transforms it into absolutely outstanding. The satisfaction in the ability to help others is the ultimate accomplishment that allows them to realize, they've really done it. They've accomplished their goal and succeeded to not only produce the outstanding results in their own life they wanted, but in others' lives as well.

Now this all looks great on paper, but I don't want to just tell you how to achieve success. I want to show you real-world examples of this powerful success formula in action so you can understand the real impact of this "success formula".

*Chapter VI*

# THE SUCCESS OF SLY

Perhaps you've heard of a man named Sylvester Stallone "Sly". Or maybe you've seen the movie Rocky? Most people have, as it won several Oscars and has been considered one of the most influential sports movies of our time.

What most don't know, is the story of how Rocky came about. How Sly made it into the movie business in the first place. And so, even though Stallone may not have known this exact "Success Formula" at the time, he definitely applied every element of it to produce the results he did. The following was taken from an interview with Stallone about his story.

Sly knew his whole life he wanted to be an actor since he was very young. He wanted to be in the movie business, period. Not TV, movies. His reason why, was that for him, it was a chance to have people not only escape, but to inspire people. And that drive is what made most of his movies.

The ability to show people what they are really capable of; inspire people to overcome unbelievable obstacles because in his own life, he felt like he did that. When he was born, he was pulled out by the forceps, that's why he looked the way he did, that's why he talked the way he did. He said, "I really wanted to do that, I knew why I wanted to do it and I wasn't willing to settle for anything else."

He knew his *Result*, and he knew the *Reason* why he wanted it.

What happened was, he went out to try and get jobs, but it's not like he went "Hey Adrian", agents went "You, you're a star!" It didn't work out so well.

He said "They looked at me and said hey you're stupid looking, do something else, you thu thu thu thu talking like this. There's no place for you in that stuff, you're never going to be a star in movies, you're insane. No one's going to want to listen to somebody who looks dopey and talks out of the side of their mouth."

And he got no after no after no. He said "I was thrown out more than 1500 times from agents' offices in New York". And there weren't 1500 agencies in New York. He had gone to some of them 5, 6, 7, 8, 9 times.

He said, one of the times "I went in to one, got in there at 4 o'clock to see one guy and he wouldn't see me, so I stayed there and wouldn't leave. I stayed overnight, he came back the next morning, and I was still sitting there. That's how I got my first job. The guy sat me down, talked to me and gave me my first movie. I was in it for about 20 seconds as the thug that somebody beat up. Because he said, people will hate your guts, you getting beat up, it'll be a good thing."

Sly did about three movies like that, never got anything, just rejection, rejection, rejection. So finally he realized it wasn't working. So he changed his approach. He said "I was starving by the way, I couldn't pay to have heat in my apartment; my wife was screaming at me every day to go get a job. But I wouldn't, because I knew that if I got a job, I'd get seduced back, and I'd lose my hunger. I knew the only way I could do this was if it was the only choice, if I'd burned all other bridges. Because if I did a normal job, pretty soon I'd be caught up in that rhythm and I'd feel okay about my life and I feel like my dream would just gradually disappear. I wanted to keep that hunger, I thought that hunger was the only thing that I had as my advantage. My wife didn't understand this at all, we got into these viscous fights."

He took *Action* and was absolutely 100% committed to achieving his vision.

So it was freezing, he was completely broke, and finally went to the public library one day because it was warm. "I didn't want to read anything, I just went in, I was hanging out there, I sat down in this chair and somebody left a book there. It was the poems of

Edgar Allen Poe. So I started reading it, and I got totally into Edgar Allen Poe. Learned everything about him, his life, his stories, his poems, and Poe got me out of myself. He got me to think about how I could touch other people, not worry about myself so much. So then I decided to become a writer."

Hard to imagine, Rocky the Writer.

He had *Result Oriented Awareness*, he was constantly evaluating what was taking him closer to his goals and what was taking him further away.

So he tried to write a bunch of screen plays, nothing worked, still totally broke, he didn't even have $50. And he said, "Finally I sold a script. It was called Paradise Alley. I sold it for $100. That $100 was a ton of money, I was so thrilled. I thought, I'm on my way!" But it never led to anything. So he kept going and going and going, finally he was so broke he hocked his wife's jewelry. He said "that was basically the end of our relationship; she hated my guts so much. Now we had nothing no food, no money, and the one thing I loved most in the world was my dog."

"I loved my dog because he gave me unconditional love, unlike my wife. What happened was, to survive, I was so broke, I couldn't feed my dog so I went to a liquor store – It was the lowest day of my life – I stood outside the liquor store trying to sell my dog to strangers. I tried to sell my dog for $50, finally one guy negotiated with me and bought my dog from me, my best friend on Earth, for $25. I walked away from there and I cried. This was the worst thing that had ever happened in my life."

Two weeks later, Sly was watching a fight between Mohamed Ali and Chuck Wepner, this white guy was getting bludgeoned but just kept on coming, and it gave Sly an idea. He said "as soon as the fight ended, I started writing. I wrote for 20 straight hours, I did not sleep. I wrote the entire movie in 20 hours straight. Right then, saw the fight, wrote the movie, whole thing, done."

"I was shaking at the end, I was so excited. I really knew, I knew what I wanted, I knew why I wanted it, I took the action, now it's time to deliver. So I went out and started trying to sell it to agents and they all would read it and say you know, this is predictable, this is stupid, this is sappy. I wrote down all the things they said and I read them the night of the Oscars when we won. The greatest revenge is massive success.

So he kept trying to sell it, he's broke, he's starving. And said "finally, I meet these guys, they read it and they believe in the script, and they love it. They offer me $125,000 for my script. I was ecstatic, but I said there's just one thing though guys, you've got a deal, but I've got to star in it. They said what are you talking about? You're a writer. I said no, no I'm an actor. They say no, no, no you're a writer. I say no, no, I'm an actor and that is my story and I am Rocky. I got to play it, I got to be the head person, I got to be the starring role."

"They said, there's no way. We're not going to pay you $125,000 take some no name and stick you in that, throw our money away. We need a star." And they wanted to have Ryan O'Neil play Rocky at the time. Sly said "no way! Ryan O'Neil isn't Rocky, I'm Rocky." Finally they said, "Well take it or leave it." He left the room and said "if that's what you believe, you don't get my script".

Now he had no money, he's totally broke, he's offered $125,000, more money than he had ever seen in his life and he walked away because he knew his real result and why he wanted it and he was committed to it. So they called him a few weeks later, and they offered him $250,000 not to star in his own movie. He turned them down; a quarter of a million dollars. They came back, there final offer was $325,000, they wanted this thing. He said, "Not without me". And they said no. Sly was totally committed to his outcome and would not settle for anything less than his true result he was after, to be a movie star.

They finally compromised in the end, and they gave him $35,000 and points in the movie because they said "If this is going to happen, then you're going to take the risk with us. And the bottom line, is we don't think it's going to work but at least we don't have to spend a bunch of money on you". They only spent $1 Million to make Rocky, and it grossed $200 Million at the time.

Here's the cool thing, $35,000 was still a lot of money when you don't even have $25. So what's the first thing Sly did with his money? Probably went out and partied or something? No.

He said, "I went to that liquor store for three straight days and hoped the man who had my dog frequented the store. I wanted to buy back my dog. Third day I was there, this guy walks by, I can't believe it, I see him and there's my dog. So I said sir, remember me? (It had been about a month and a half). Remember me? I'm the guy who sold you the dog." Sly continued, "he said yeah, yeah I love the dog. I said look, I was so broke, I was starving, he's my best friend, I'm sure you love him too but I got to have him back. Please, I beg of you. I'll pay you $100 for the dog. I know I gave him to you for $25, I'll give you $100. The man said absolutely not, no way. He's my dog now, you can't buy him back. So I offered him $500 for the dog. The guy said absolutely not, no way. $1000 for my dog. The guy said no amount of money on Earth is ever going to get this dog from me!"

Sly knew his outcome though and he was committed so in the end, he finally got his dog. He knew his result, took action and just changed his approach until he got it. $15,000 and a part in Rocky, is what it took for him to get his dog back. The dog in Rocky, Buttkiss, is Sly's real dog. He put his dog in the movie, he put the guy in the movie and paid $15,000 when he was only paid $35,000 for the movie.

Isn't that pretty awesome? I thought that was such a cool thing.

He *Changed his Approach* until he succeeded, and *Gave Back* to the world by inspiring millions with his inspirational movies.

Clearly, Sly is a guy who understands the formula for success. Because he never gave up, he kept taking action and changing his approach and was so focused on his vision, he was able to accomplish greater success than most could ever dream of.

That is the power of this incredible formula. And that is what sets the super achievers apart from the rest of society.

So that's one example of how the success formula was applied in real life to accomplish something incredible. But that was for the movie business. You might be wondering though, can this same formula be applied to achieve success in fitness and other areas of your life as well?

## *Chapter VII*
# SUCCESSINATOR

To answer this, I want to share the story of one of the most influential individuals in the history of the fitness industry, Arnold Schwarzenegger. Even "The Governator" himself used the principles of this incredibly powerful formula to achieve ultimate success in not only his fitness and health, but also in acting and politics. He achieved greater success in three separate careers than most individuals achieve in either one in their lifetime. And he did it by applying these same principles of the success formula.

To illustrate his story, the following was pulled from a biography documentary and Arnold's commencement speech at the University of Southern California:

Arnold was brought up very strict in a little village (Thal, Austria). His father was a police officer, and "wanted him to go to the military and marry a Heidi or a Grettle with braids and to be happy ever after" according to Arnold.

Early in Arnold's life he discovered he thought very differently from the rest of the people he grew up with.

He said, "in Austria kids were conditioned to follow their parent's path. But unlike other kids around me, I was very determined that I have to get out of there. And then one day, I saw the cover of a magazine with Reg Park and it says 'How Mr. Universe became Hercules'. I opened up this magazine and I read through it and there was the whole plan laid out".

Arnold found his *vision* and a plan to make it possible.

But back then, bodybuilding did not exist in Austria. His friends would constantly mock him saying "come on Arnold. You're dreaming. Give it up!" And his father didn't like it at all.

Arnold recounted, "My father, he said this is an embarrassment to me, and was stomping all over me, so in 1965, at the age of 18, he got me set up with his pals in the military to become a tank driver. But I was talking about becoming the most muscular man in the world. The problem was how do I go now and train every day in the military base? I said to myself, Okay Arnold, here's the goal and whatever it takes to get there, I will do".

He knew his *Result*! He had a vivid, clear picture of exactly what he wanted to accomplish, being the most muscular man in the world.

He continued, "So I was doing my daily work, cleaning the guns and going to the shooting range, marching 20 miles a day and crawling around up hills with weapons, running at 5 in the morning in heavy combat boots and all of this stuff. And then everyone just almost drops dead at night, is totally exhausted. I worked out 3 hours and got up early in the morning again to do my sit ups and my push ups and my chin ups."

Arnold was absolutely committed to his end-result and did more than anyone else would ever expect in order to keep moving towards success.

He continued, "There was a clear conflict, a dilemma because the lifting wasn't a traditional sport for them. They didn't like the idea, they didn't even have the equipment. I had to go and figure out every way possible, I'd do dips between chairs, or put a bar across two chairs and do upside down rowing".

"Everyone would say this is the wrong direction that I'm going, or I'm in a dream world, that I'm useless. Whatever it was, I said, I'm going to break through that. No matter what it takes, I needed to reach that goal, that vision that I had of being a world champion".

He had a blueprint and *strategy* to get to his goal and he took consistent *action*, every single day to get him closer to his *vision*! He was committed to doing whatever it took, no matter what. He used every resource he could think of to keep stepping closer to his goal, finding ways to continue working out even when there was no traditional equipment there for him to train with.

Then one week, he got an invitation to go to the Junior Mr. Europe Bodybuilding Championship. "Here's an international competition and if I really wanted to start making a big splash, that competition was the way to go. A year later, I couldn't have entered because if you get past 18, then you're not allowed to compete anymore. So I said Oh my God. How am I going to get out of here to go to this competition? I'm going through basic training. And if I leave, the consequences were severe" He pondered. Those who left without permission were sent to solitary confinement which could be several days or several weeks.

"I was lying in bed and questioning myself, do you really want that Arnold? If they put me in jail, what does that mean about me? I had my doubts. In the meantime, time was running out, the bodybuilding competition was approaching very quickly. This caused me sleepless nights.

I asked myself, Arnold what is it about you that is so different? Why are you the only one that sees it so clearly, this goal, going to America and winning the Mr. Universe contest and getting into movies, and making millions of dollars? No one else talks about this around here. Is it real? Is it just a crazy fantasy? But, wait a minute, Reg Park did it, then it's possible. Arnold, focus, the key thing is to be focused; visualize your goal. And I saw myself standing up there on stage, just like Reg Park and it became more and more clear, Arnold, you've got to go".

He had *Result Oriented Awareness*. He was constantly evaluating what would get him closer to his goal and what would not.

The most difficult part was, how to get to the competition when he was not supposed to leave the country. And the answer was freight trains, they didn't stop at the border so he could get there without being found. It took a minimum of 26 hours, when it normally takes 5 hours. So that's what he did.

Finally he arrived there the afternoon of the competition and didn't have anything with him, not even gym clothes. So he said "I had to go and find someone from the lighter weight category, he was finished with the posing, and I asked him for his trunks. They were all schmutzed, you can imagine. So I took his trunks and went out and my posing was very clumsy. But then I got called out again on stage and again on stage, and I felt more and more confident that I'm in the top 3 because every time I posed, there was much more applause. So I started playing to the audience, I'm the young guy, the new guy on the block.

Sure enough, they announced number 3, number 2, and I was the winner. I just couldn't believe it. It was one of those important moments because I realized that I was not dreaming. They've never heard of me, and they picked me, so I must have something that is unique".

When Arnold went back to training, he couldn't just walk back in through the gates and say "Hi, I'm back". So he found another place where he could sneak back in. He said, "The idea was to just melt back into the room where you're part of the daily activities. It didn't work", he laughed. "They have good guarding, so that's the way I got caught. I had to spend several days in solitary confinement which was the punishment".

But he reminded himself, "Yes it's painful, yes it's going to hurt, but look at the consequences, it doesn't scare me. Your overall goal is not to create a career here in the military. They will stifle you, they will hold you back for the rest of your life; the key thing is to not let your eye off that vision". Finally they wanted to meet with him in the Lieutenant's office. There was 3 or 4 officers there and they started really harsh, screaming at Arnold. "How could you do this to us? You violated the rules". Arnold apologized profusely, and then eventually the whole thing settled down.

He recounted, "Somehow, the word got around that I won. And they said, let's get this straight, that you won the competition?" He gave them credit right away and said, "It's because I had the opportunity to train, running and climbing and crawling up the hills with the gun in my hand". And they said, "That's good right guys?" They all kind of agreed, because in the military they love discipline. So they loved using Arnold as an example after that. They were very proud, but at the same time, they had to do something, officially. So they said "We're going to punish you Schwarzenegger... and send you into the kitchen to peel the potatoes".

Arnold joyfully mentioned "So then I got my extra food, they slapped on an extra steak. It was the first time I had meat and had protein every day. Then all the welders got together and built machines and equipment and the Lieutenants ensured that I could train every day from 3 til 6. I had my portable gym for when we were sent into the desert, we put all this equipment in the tank and so we were prepared at any given time and we trained".

He *Changed his Approach*, overcoming every obstacle that came his way to keep progressing towards his dream.

He elated, "It was a perfect marriage, because they needed me, and I definitely needed them. Before, I felt like I was struggling on my own and all of a sudden it felt like there was a team around me. During that year that I spent there, I gained literally 25lbs of solid muscle. That year, the base paved the way for the future".

Arnold used the success formula to become one of the greatest bodybuilders of all time and one of the most influential individuals in the fitness industry. He also *Gave Back* through inspiring millions with his accomplishments and motivating young hopefuls all around the world wishing to make it in bodybuilding. But Arnold didn't just apply the success formula to this one area of his life, he applied it to every area.

When he wanted to get into acting, people said "No, you have an accent and a body that is too big, a name no one can pronounce; be realistic. It is the 70s, today Dustin Hoffman, he is the big shot, Al Pacino, little guys, Woody Allen, sex symbol". But Arnold went on to be the highest grossing action star in the movie business. He achieved truly outstanding success, more than anyone else ever had by having a clear understanding of the key to success and consistently taking action.

Arnold went on to inspire millions more with his acting, then wanted to find more ways to give back and eventually got into politics.

He mentioned, "Even when I ran for Governor, they said are you kidding me? You can never win, give it up! But I didn't pay any attention because I said to myself, what if I do? When they said you can't go to Germany, you can't compete in the Junior Mr. Europe, I did not listen to the no. I went and it worked out. And I used that attitude as a blueprint for the rest of my life".

Arnold's success in so many areas of his life all comes back to his ability to consistently take action towards his dreams and goals. He truly exemplifies the extraordinary possibilities of applying this success formula to your own life.

Now, Arnold did not necessarily know this exact formula at the time, he had his own rules for success that he followed, which I'll share with you here. But I think you'll find, even though his rules are slightly different, they still follow the same ultimate formula and the one key that made it all possible was *consistent action*.

So here are Arnold's 6 Rules for Success as he shared them at his address at the 2009 USC Commencement:

1. **Trust Yourself**

He said you have to "dig deep down and ask yourselves who do you want to be? Not what, but who? Not what your parents and teachers want you to be; you". You have to figure out for yourselves what makes you happy, no matter how crazy it sounds to other people.

2. **Break The Rules**

There are so many rules in life about everything, Arnold says "break the rules, not the law but break the rules. It is impossible to be a maverick or a true original if you're too well behaved and don't want to break the rules. You have to think outside the box. After all, what is the point of being on this Earth if all you want to be is liked by everyone and avoid trouble? The only way I ever got any place was by breaking some of the rules".

3. **Don't Be Afraid To Fail**

Arnold mentioned he was always willing to fail at everything he ever attempted. "You can't always win but don't be afraid of making decisions. You can't be paralyzed by fear of failure or you will never push yourself. You keep pushing because you believe in yourself and your vision and you know that it's the right thing to do. Success will come, so don't be afraid to fail".

4. **Don't Listen to the Nay-sayers**

He asked "How many times have you heard you can't do this? Or you can't do that? It has never been done before". He heard this all the time and he loved it when someone said "No one has ever done this before" because he stated "Then I do it, that means that I am the first that has done it. So pay no attention to the people who say it can't be done".

5. **Work Your Butt Off**

This Arnold mentions is the most important rule of all. "You never want to fail because you didn't work hard enough. I never want to lose a competition because I didn't work hard enough. I always believed leaving no stone un-turned. Mohamad Ali, one of my great heroes, had a great line in the 70s when he was asked, how many sit-ups do you do? He said I don't count my sit-ups, I only start counting when it starts hurting, when I feel pain, because that's when it really counts, that's what makes you a champion, that's the way it is with everything. No pain, no gain." He continues "If you want to coast through life, don't pay any attention to these rules but if you want to win there's absolutely no way around it, hard, hard work. I've always figured out, there's 24 hours in a day, you sleep 6 hours, and you have 18 hours left. – now I know there's some of you out there now that say well wait a minute, I sleep 8 hours or 9 hours; well then just sleep faster, I would recommend. Because you only need to sleep 6 hours, you have 18 hours left and there's a lot of things you can accomplish. Just remember, you can't climb the ladder of success with your hands in the pocket".

## 6. **Give Back**

Arnold also believed in contributing back to others. "Whatever path you take in your lives, you must always find time to give something back. Something back to your community, give something back to your state or your country. Tear down that mirror. Tear down that mirror that makes you always look at yourself. And you will be able to look beyond that mirror and you will see the millions of people that need your help. Let me tell you something, reaching out and helping people will bring you more satisfaction than anything else you've ever done".

These are a great set of rules to follow and include in your life and I believe they really mesh perfectly with our powerful success formula.

So I hope you can see the true power and magnitude of the possibilities with this formula. And now I want to make sure you are able to use it. So let's really put this into action for ourselves right now and apply it to our health and fitness.

*Chapter VIII*
# BUILDING THE BLUEPRINT

The very first thing before anything else is that you have to have a vision. You have to have a clear, precise, focused vision of exactly what it is you want to achieve. For anything great I've ever achieved in my life, it always started with a clear vision of exactly how I wanted it to be, with so much power, so much emotion that I could feel exactly how it would feel when it came true. And that vision is what kept me focused on my result. It was compelling enough to literally pull me towards it through all the times when things got tough, just like in the success formula and in the examples we discussed above.

So the first step is to create a **vision** for what you want to achieve. And I don't just want you to picture some skinny person if your goal is to lose weight. I want you to see yourself at your ideal weight. I want you to feel the feelings you would feel when you reached your goal, say the things you'd be saying to yourself when you achieved that goal and really feel as though it has already come true.

Right now, I want you to take 5-10 minutes and really get a clear vision of what you want to accomplish in your fitness and health. Close your eyes and picture your dream body; you want to be strong? You're strong! You want to have chiseled 6-pack abs? You've got that washboard! Picture everything you can, stand right now how you would be standing if you had your dream body right now. Make the facial expression you'd have when you achieved your ultimate physique. Breathe how you would be breathing if you were totally healthy, fit and strong. Feel how you'd be feeling if you were at your absolute peak level of fitness and health! What sort of things can you do now that you never could before? Are you more flexible? Are you vibrant and full of energy? Are you strong and powerful? What else could you do? What would you be saying to yourself in your head, accomplishing your dream body?

This is who you are, who you were always meant to be. What you always knew you could be! Now, in this peak state, feeling and breathing and seeing everything exactly how you've always wanted it to be. I want you to write out every detail about this experience so you have a clear description of exactly what your vision is.

Write out **'*My Ultimate Vision*'** or visit: **www.IIFYMbook.com/Success-Section** for a free printable PDF **Success Workbook**, and start writing down how you look, how you feel, how confident you are, how strong or powerful or vibrant, all the new things you can accomplish as this person, all the things you say to yourself as this person, get it all down. This is your dream, nobody else's. Everything you need to accomplish this is already inside you.

Got it all? Fantastic! Let's keep things rolling!

Now that you've gotten that written out, you have a complete description of exactly what your vision is for your dream results! And by seeing and feeling as though you've already achieved your goal, you are sending powerful signals to your subconscious mind and firing up your brain to start moving you towards it. So that is the first part of step one.

The next thing you must do if you really want to achieve your goal, is you have to develop a strong enough **reason** for **why** you want it. Why some people fail in spite of every opportunity and others achieve in spite of every obstacle, I believe is driven from their reason or lack of reason why they want to achieve their goal. If you have a strong enough reason why you must accomplish something, you will find a way to make it happen, no matter what it takes.

If your reason is powerful enough and meaningful enough to you, nothing can stop you from achieving your goal. You will run through walls to get to what you want. But if you don't have a strong enough reason why you want to accomplish something, then at the slightest set back, you're just going to give up.

So now that you have your ultimate vision, I want you to write down why you absolutely **MUST** achieve this goal. Not why you should, not why you could, not why you ought to, why you **MUST** accomplish this. Write down all the pain that you have right now by not having accomplished your ultimate vision. What are you not able to do now that you could if you had accomplished your ultimate vision? How would you feel going through another year without getting any closer to your goal? 3 years? 5 years without any progress toward your goal? My hallucination is pretty lousy right? Write it down. Be real with yourself. We have to create that strong reason that forces you into action and change!

Now write down all the pleasure you would gain from accomplishing your ultimate vision. Knowing every single day you were doing something to bring you one step closer to your ultimate vision. Why do you want it? What will it give you? Will you be more confident? Will you have more to give to others? Will you be a better role model for someone, a child, a sibling? Why will you do whatever it takes to accomplish your goal? Why will you absolutely make this happen no matter what? What is it that causes that burning desire within you, that will excite you and get your blood pumping every time you think of it? Write every reason you can think of down right now.

Doesn't that feel incredible?

Perfect! You now have your ***ultimate vision*** of your goal and the powerful driving ***reason*** behind why you must accomplish it. You are well on your way to ultimate success! Step one complete!

Next is step two. You have your *what*, you have your *why*, now it's time to develop your *way forward*. Now that you have your vision and you know exactly why you want it so bad, the next thing to do is develop a ***strategy*** to get you there. So let's do it!

It is okay if you don't have all the pieces of the puzzle figured out yet, this does not have to be perfect. One of the biggest mistakes people make when trying to create their plan for success, is they try to make everything perfect before they take action. I've got news for you though. Nothing is perfect. Perfect is a low standard. If you try to set yourself up for perfection, you are always setting yourself up for failure. And this is the reason so many people get stopped on their path to success before they ever even get started. They get caught up trying to create the perfect plan and never end up taking any action because their plan isn't quite perfect enough yet. This is why so many people get stuck merely having a dream and never making it a reality. If you wait for all the lights on the road to be green before heading out, you'll never be able to leave your driveway. So throw out that word perfect and let's get to taking action!

Right now, I want you to write out *10 different ways* you can get just one single step closer to your ultimate goal. There are a million and one ways to make a million dollars but not all of them work for every person. So you have 5 minutes right now, write down 10 different tiny, simple steps you can take immediately to move you one step closer to your ultimate goal. Don't over-complicate this; these should be simple steps you can immediately take action on. Could you visit a local gym and ask about a membership? Could you hire a personal trainer or coach to help you out? Could you go for a jog in the park? What are some simple actionable steps you can take to move yourself one step closer to your goal? Could you call a friend and schedule a workout? Could you go play a game of basketball or go for a hike? What simple thing could you do right now? Got all 10? Awesome!

Now it's time to take **action**! Choose **one** of the steps you just wrote down and **do not continue reading this book until you have taken action on it**. I'm serious. Do not put this off any longer. Remember the key difference that separates the successful from the rest of the world? Taking consistent **action**. So stop reading this book right now until you have taken action on at least one of your action steps! Do it now!

Welcome back! Did you do your homework? Did you take your first action step towards your ultimate vision? If not, go back and do it right now!

If you did though, I want to congratulate you! You have just taken your first step towards ultimate success and achieving your dream. You are now one step closer than you were before, and one step closer than all the millions of other people who are still stuck at the stage of merely having a dream. You are 10 x further ahead than the 99% of people who still haven't taken that first step!

That's really all it takes. All you have to do to accomplish any dream you ever have, is to consistently take one simple step at a time to move you closer to achieving it. Every action you take builds on the action before it and every step forward builds momentum, making the next one easier and easier.

That is how all of the most successful people in the world achieve excellence in any area of their life. Commit to consistently take action, no matter what! You must absolutely 100% commit to taking these simple action steps, no matter how trivial or complicated they may seem at the time. Only through those consistent actions can you get to your ultimate destination.

Now the third step in the formula for success is to have **Result Oriented Awareness** or **ROA**. ROA is a continual process that you must stick with. Every action step you take and every result you produce, you have to decide whether it is taking you closer to or further away from your *ultimate vision*. Whether you fail or succeed, always be aware of the results you're producing from the actions you're taking and notice whether you're on track, or off track.

The fourth step then, is to **change your approach**. There will be hard times that arise. You will make mistakes, everyone does. The difference though that sets the achievers apart from the non-achievers is how they handle these set-backs.

The super successful have a different definition and response to failure that allows them to keep moving forward. If they fail at one thing, they use their *ROA*, determine why they "failed" and *change their approach*. They take a new *action* to produce a new result and continue moving towards their goal. They do not get all strung up on failures and label themselves as failures. They simply acknowledge the fact that they failed at doing something, and figure out a new action step to take them one step closer to their *ultimate vision* again.

If you apply these four steps to your life, you create your **ultimate vision**, define your **why**, you develop a **strategy** with simple action steps to take you one step closer to your dream; and you commit to take **consistent action** with them, you are aware of the results you're producing and the **direction** they're taking you and you continually **change your approach** to keep progressing towards your dreams, I guarantee you will create greater success and achievement in any area of your life than ever before. You will be able to accomplish far more than you ever thought possible and you will create your ultimate dream physique.

Finally, once you've accomplished success in your own life, the fifth and final step to ultimate success and achievement is to find a way to **give back**. If you managed to lose weight and maintain a new healthy lifestyle, maybe you can help a friend accomplish the same? If you have a success story that would inspire others to take action, maybe you can share it with friends and family or post a blog or video about it. If this book helped you achieve more in your life, perhaps there is someone else in your life who could benefit from reading this book? Whatever it is, if you can find a way to *give back* and contribute to others,; I promise you will receive a level of satisfaction like you've never felt before!

Okay, I know this was a long section, and I'm so glad you've made it through. Because I think this is one of the most important sections in this entire book! Many other books will explain what you should do and what you could do, but hardly any actually take the time to really walk you through the actions to make a real change.

I believe this is one of the key areas that sets this book apart from all the other health and fitness books out there. This is not just some informational book on what to eat and what not to eat. This is a guide to ensure you have every resource available to achieve your ultimate goals. Whether you want to know how to lose weight, how to build muscle, how to lose fat, how to maintain a healthy lifestyle, or how to achieve an incredible looking physique, I want this to allow you to achieve ultimate success with that goal. This book is meant to literally guide you along your journey to success.

Again, this section, although long, was just an introduction to the ultimate success and achievement you can attain through health, fitness and any other area of your life. This is covered in full depth and detail in my book on Ultimate Fitness Lifestyle Success at:
**www.IIFYMbook.com/Success-Book** if you would really like to take this to the next level.

Now that you're set up for success, it's time to move on to the final section! It's time to get started on IIFYM or Flexible Dieting!

## *Chapter IX*
# GETTING STARTED

Okay, I'm starting to believe… How the heck do I start?

Well, now you know what Flexible Dieting is, how general weight loss works, how your body composition is effected by the macronutrients you consume and why flexible dieting can be a more effective and enjoyable approach to a healthier lifestyle than traditional rigid approaches. You also have your ultimate vision, and your strategy for ultimate success.

So now it's time to dive right in and get started on your own transformation to truly achieve the body of your dreams, to Engineer your Alpha Physique! It's time to look your best, do your best and BE your best!

*Chapter X*

# STEP ONE –
# CALCULATE CALORIES

In order to get started with Flexible Dieting, the first thing to figure out is how many calories you should eat each day, whether you're looking to burn body fat or build solid lean muscle mass.

Now there are a lot of free online calculators you may use to figure out your daily caloric maintenance level; this is, the amount of calories you must eat each day to maintain your exact body weight you are at now.

You can also calculate maintenance calorie level yourself using any of the three following methods:

**A.** The Basic Multiplier (*least accurate*)
**B.** The Harris-Benedict Formula (*more accurate*)
**C.** The Katch-McArdle Formula (*most accurate*)

## A. The Basic Multiplier

Although this is a very straightforward and basic method, in the majority of situations it will work just fine for average trainees with average body types.

The Basic Multiplier is simply a matter of multiplying your current bodyweight (in pounds) by a set number. To maintain your current body weight, this usually means around 14-16.

### Your bodyweight x 14-16

So if you weigh 180lbs, it would look like this…
**180 x 14 = 2520**
**180 x 16 = 2880**
Daily caloric intake should be **2520-2880** calories.

Now to *lose weight* you will subtract **300-500** calories from your caloric maintenance level.

To *gain weight* you will add **300-500** calories to your caloric maintenance level.

This will allow you to *burn* or *build* approximately **0.5-1lb/week** which is a healthy rate.

The drawback to this method is that it doesn't take into account individual factors such as lean body mass, height, sex or activity level. For those who do not have an "average" build (starting more on the overweight side or more muscular side) and who do not have "average" activity levels, methods B and C will be more accurate.

For average trainees with average body weight and activity levels, this method will usually work fine.


## B. The Harris Benedict Formula

This is the second most accurate method and is superior to the Basic Multiplier because it takes height, sex, age and activity level into account on top of your basic bodyweight.

The first goal with this method is to determine your **Basal Metabolic Rate (BMR)**. Your basal metabolic rate is the total number of calories that your body requires to perform all of its natural daily functions. This does not include extra activities such as weight training or playing sports; the BMR is for natural processes such as breathing, digesting food, regulating body temperature etc.

Once you have figured out your BMR, you can then plug it into the **Activity Multiplier** (how active you are on a daily basis) in order to determine your **Caloric Maintenance Level**.

## Calculating the Harris-Benedict Formula

| 1KG | = 2.2Lbs |
|------|-----------|
| 1 IN | = 2.54cm |

### Calculating Basal Metabolic Rate
**Men: 66 + (13.7 X bodyweight in kg) + (5 X height in cm) - (6.8 X age in years)**

**Women: 655 + (9.6 X bodyweight in kg) + (1.8 X height in cm) - (4.7 X age in years)**

Take that number and multiply it by...

### Activity Multiplier
- **Sedentary** = BMR X **1.2** (little to no exercise)
- **Lightly Active** = BMR X **1.375** (light exercise: 1-3 days a week)
- **Moderately Active** = BMR X **1.55** (moderate exercise: 3-5 days a week)
- **Very Active** = BMR X **1.725** (intense exercise: 6-7 days a week)
- **Extremely Active** = BMR X **1.9** (intense daily exercise and strenuous physical job)

This will give you your caloric maintenance level. Again you will want to take that number and add or subtract 300-500 calories to find your daily caloric intake for gaining or losing weight.

### Example of the Harris Benedict Formula:
In case you're a bit confused, here is an example of how to plug all of this information in.

Take Joe as our example. Joe weighs **82kg**, he is **177.8cm** tall, he's **25 years old** and **moderately active**.

First we determine Joe's Basal Metabolic Rate...
**BMR = 66 + 1123.4 + 889 – 170 = 1908**

Joes Basal Metabolic Rate is **1908 calories.** This is the number of calories that he requires daily in order for his normal bodily processes to be carried out. We'll now take his activity level into account by multiplying his BMR by the appropriate activity multiplier.

**1908 (BMR) x 1.55 (Moderate Activity) = 2957.4**

This means that Joes needs to consume **2957 calories** per day in order to *maintain* his weight. In order to create a caloric deficit that supports fat loss or a caloric surplus that supports muscle growth, he needs to subtract or add 300-500 calories to his maintenance level.

**2957 – 300 = 2657**
**2957 – 500 = 2457**

Joe's daily intake should be **2457-2657 calories** to lose weight.

## C. The Katch-McArdle Formula

This is the most accurate formula of all because it takes into account the specific individual factor of *lean body mass*, and this will result in a more accurate Basal Metabolic Rate reading.

The Harris-Benedict formula outlined on the previous pages is a great method and will be accurate in almost all situations, but still has one drawback in that it doesn't take lean body mass into account.

This is fine for most people, but for those who have a high amount of body fat or a high amount of muscle it will not be as accurate.

If you've had your lean body mass tested (testing lean body mass is beyond the scope of this book, and there are a ton of different methods used for this) then you can use the following formula to get the most accurate reading of all.

**BMR = 370 + (21.6 X lean mass in kg)**

You can then multiply your BMR by the Activity Multiplier in order to figure out your caloric maintenance level. (Refer back to the Harris-Benedict formula for the activity multiplier)

You should then add/ subtract **300-500** calories to that number in order to figure out your daily caloric intake for weight gain or weight loss.

It's really as simple as that.

*Chapter XI*
# STEP TWO –
# CALCULATE MACRO RATIOS

Now, once you've calculated your daily caloric intake for either gaining or losing weight. The next step in the process is to figure out the macronutrient ratio you need to build muscle or burn body fat.

This step is the most crucial in improving your overall body composition and really achieving your dream body and it is also extremely specific to each individual.

Here are a few macro ratios of some of the popular diets by percentages to give you an idea (%Carb: %Protein: %Fat):

- *Traditional Bodybuilding Diet* (45:35:20)
- *The Zone Diet* (40:30:30)
- *Ketogenic Diet* (10:45:45)
- *South Beach Diet* (28:33:39)
- *Atkins Diet* (6:35:59)
- *Protein Power Diet* (9:37:54)

As you can see there are a lot of variations from diet to diet and no one approach is best over all others. Every *body* responds differently and the ratio you follow will also depend largely on your fitness and health goals and what you're looking to accomplish.

So you may be wondering, how do I know what macronutrient ratio to start out with or what would be right for me?

First, if you're just getting started, I would recommend sticking with a more *moderate, well balanced ratio*. With a well-balanced macro ratio you can achieve fat loss and muscle growth and get some great results without compromising your overall health;

Perhaps you could try something along the lines of 35% Carbs: 35% Protein: 30% Fat, just for example.

Note: If you would like to know a little more about how to choose a good starting macro ratio for yourself based on your fitness and health goals, refer to the bonus chapter "*Making the Most of Macros*" on **page 60** at the end of this step!

Otherwise, if you're happy starting out with a balanced ratio or you find one of the ratios such as the *Traditional Bodybuilding Diet* suits your goals, you can skip right by the bonus-section and continue on with the next action steps to get started right away!

Now to clarify, let's use the example of our good buddy Joe from above who is **180lbs,** and wants to achieve a healthy rate of weight loss at **1lb** per week. Joe also follows a bodybuilding style of exercise routine.

So in this case, we will use the *Traditional Bodybuilding* macronutrient ratio for this.
We already know that in order for Joe to lose **1lb/week**, he needs to consume **2457 calories**.

In order to ensure Joe is losing *body fat* for that **1lb loss** per week, we need to make sure he's following his macronutrient ratios properly for his 2457 calorie budget.

So we take his daily caloric intake for fat loss **2457 calories,** and use the ratio (**45:35:20**) to figure out how many calories he needs to consume of each macronutrient.

| | | |
|---|---|---|
| **45% Carbohydrate** | **(2457 x 0.45)** | **= 1106 Calories** |
| **35% Protein** | **(2457 x 0.35)** | **= 860 Calories** |
| **20% Fat** | **(2457 x 0.20)** | **= 491 Calories** |

This gives Joe the amount of **calories** to consume of each macronutrient but we're not done yet. Now we have to figure out how many **grams** of each will give him those calories to make it easy for him to track his macros using nutrition information and food databases.

So we know from the beginning of the book, each macronutrient has a caloric value:

| | |
|---|---|
| **1 gram protein** | **= 4 calories** |
| **1 gram carbohydrate** | **= 4 calories** |
| **1 gram fat** | **= 9 calories** |

Now we simply divide the **calories** for each macro by the number of **calories per gram** in each, to get the **gram** amounts of each macronutrient:

**45% Carbohydrate**    (1106 / 4)        = 276.5g

**35% Protein**        (860 / 4)        = 215g

**20% Fat**        (491 / 9)        = 54.5g

Therefore Joe needs to consume **276.5g Carbs**, **215g Protein**, and **54.5g Fats** daily in order to achieve his goal of losing **1lb** of **body fat** per week.

It's as easy as that!

Now these percentage ratios are really just an introductory starting point for flexible dieting. This is a great way for you to get started with flexible dieting and you can absolutely achieve incredible results just by following these guidelines and using percentage macro ratios. However, as the body composition changes and responds differently over time it becomes more and more important to base amounts of each macronutrient on your individual body, insulin response, your fitness goals and simply how your body responds to certain foods.

Additionally, to improve results and keep things progressing without running into "plateaus", more advanced principles and techniques such as carb cycling and structured refeeds should be introduced into the diet for a complete plan. These serve many crucial steps to achieving the most effective and maintainable results possible. These additional principles help with boosting your metabolism, curbing hunger levels or cravings, ensuring you have sufficient energy, ensuring you maintain your strength and more. However these are beyond the scope of this book as they require very specific and individual attention.

Therefore, in order to get the absolute most out your macros and your fitness and nutrition goals you should seek the help of a professional. If you would like help from yours truly, "*The APE Coach*", to really get the most out of your training and nutrition, you can apply to my exclusive online coaching program at (www.APEcoach.com/Coaching) for a complete individualized plan and ongoing coaching and program adjustments directly from me.

*Please note, due to high demand and my focus on providing the best possible service to each and every client I work with, not everyone may be accepted for the program. But I'd love to hear from you and I will be in touch with you regardless.*

## *Chapter XII*
# BONUS –
# MAKING THE MOST OF MACROS

Alright, so you're understanding how to calculate your daily calorie intake based on your goals, and now how to figure out your macros for that calorie amount. But you want to know more about making the most of your macros and how you can get started with a better macro ratio for your needs and goals.

In this section, I'll share some general guidelines to point you in the right direction towards choosing your starting macro ratio.

Again, my goal with this book is not to overload you with information, or impress you with my vast knowledge. In today's day and age, we are drowning in information and what we're really starving for is how to use it!

So my goal with this book is to keep things as simple as possible, and provide you with just the information necessary to allow you to take action and achieve results. I want you to be able to read this book, understand the information, and immediately be able to apply the simple action steps in your life to start producing life-transforming results!

So without boring you on the details of all the different energy systems within our body, or how the body processes each macronutrient to produce energy for different purposes, I simply want to explain to you and show you what macros you should focus on more, based on the types of activities and physical demands you have.

For simplicity's sake we will divide individuals in to 3 classes based on type of activity:

**CLASS A)** Mostly High Intensity, Explosive, Strength or Power activities/exercise.

**CLASS B)** Mostly Lower Intensity, Endurance activities/exercise.

**CLASS C)** Sedentary, Little to no activity/exercise.

Now based, on these classes, each will have a dominant energy system that fuels them during their activities/exercise; mainly carbohydrates, fat or both.

However, before I dive into each class, I want to mention that protein should always be given high priority no matter what class of activity/exercise you may fall under.

Protein is very important for recovery, strength and improving lean body mass no matter your activity/exercise types or levels. With that being said, let's look at the classes now.

### Class A (i.e. Bodybuilders, Powerlifters and those in High Intensity Sports)

The type of exercise and activity Class A individuals partake in requires a higher demand for carbohydrates to fuel their body. Therefore, a ratio similar to the *Traditional Bodybuilding Diet* (45% Carbs: 35% Protein: 20% Fat) that emphasizes the majority of macros around carbs would be best suited for these individuals.

### Class B (i.e. Walkers, Long Distance Joggers, Marathoners, and those in Endurance Sports)

The type of exercise and activity Class B individuals partake in requires a higher demand for fats to fuel their body. Therefore, a ratio such as the *South Beach Diet* (28% Carbs: 33% Protein: 39% Fats) or the *Ketogenic Diet* (10% Carbs: 45% Protein: 45% Fats) that emphasizes the majority of macros around fats would be best suited for these individuals.

However, personally I do not like going to the extreme ends of dropping any one particular macronutrient below 15-20% as all three macronutrients are important in maintaining a healthy lifestyle overall.

## Class C (i.e. People who do little to no physical activity or exercise)

Let me just say, if you are not doing any physical activity or exercise, it would be very wise to start. Along with looking better and improving your fitness, exercise and physical activity can be beneficial in so many ways for maintaining a healthy lifestyle. From physical, to emotional and psychological well-being, as well as the prevention and improvements of countless disorders and diseases, it is a no-brainer. Plus it's easy to start!

Just like this book shows you, proper nutrition and dieting to achieve your dream body doesn't have to be so difficult; exercise is the exact same.

Whether you've got a couple hours a day that you could work in some exercise or you've only got 90mins of down time in the entire week; you can start an exercise routine and achieve incredible results. That is all it takes to really produce life-changing results in your health and fitness, especially when combined with the information on nutrition in this book!

While you can achieve incredible results in your health and your body from nutrition alone, physical exercise is crucial to creating and maintaining a well-balanced, healthy lifestyle. And if you can't work in just 90 minutes out of a whole week, perhaps it's time to re-evaluate some things in your life or you may not be around to enjoy much more of it…

So if you need help getting started, please contact me. I will gladly work with you to design a routine that completely fits your needs and your busy lifestyle!

That being said, if you currently are inactive or only do a little physical activity here and there, it would be best to stick with a well-balanced macro ratio such as the (35% Carbs: 35% Protein: 30% Fat) ratio mentioned earlier.

So there you have it, I hope you've got a better understanding of the proper macronutrient ratios for you and your goals now. Time to move on the next step and *really* make the most of your macros by getting started today!

*Chapter XIII*

# STEP THREE –
# GET A MACRO TRACKER

This approach to eating is all about tracking and measuring your macronutrient intake. Getting a macro-tracking app such as LoseIt or MyFitnessPal will allow you to easily track the macros in the foods you eat. They are both free and work across all platforms. They also both have all the information on how to track your foods and how the apps work on their site, so you can easily read through and learn how to use them effectively.

Personally I use 'LoseIt' as I find it to be the most user friendly, the easiest to add custom foods and just like the layout the most of all the apps I've tried. But whatever you find works best for you is what you should go with. The idea is to make it as easy and convenient as possible for you to keep track of your macros so that you're more likely to do it consistently. Remember, your brain is always trying to seek pleasure and avoid pain, so the less painful you can make it for yourself the better you'll do!

Having the macro-tracking app makes life a lot easier when it comes to keeping track of your diet!

For starters, these apps both have a large food database included in the app; so the majority of foods you can quickly search for and find all of the nutrition info you need! These food databases include a ton of your regular grocery items and also include many restaurants and fast food joints as well. This arms you with the ability to stick to your macros no matter where you are or what you're having.

Second, they include a barcode scanner, so if you have a specific brand of food, or anything with a barcode on it, you just scan it and presto! It gives you all the nutrition info for that food. Finally, if the food doesn't scan in or you can't seem to find it on the database, you can easily enter your own custom foods into the app and even create your own recipes and share with friends.

Save yourself the headache and manual labour of reading every single nutrition label and looking up nutrition facts for foods online and writing everything out by hand. That is too time consuming to stick to long term and just a royal pain! Get a macro tracking app and get started using it right away. This will be your new best friend and make tracking your food a breeze! It takes about 30 seconds to search for and download one of these apps on your phone so do it right now, I'll wait... Got it? Good!

Now that you've got your app it's time to start tracking your foods and hitting your goal daily macro amounts that you calculated in the previous step! Let's go back to our good friend Joe. If you recall, Joe's goal macronutrient amounts for each day are **276.5g carbs, 215g protein** and **54.5g fat**. So Joe's goal is to track his food and drinks and by the end of the day have the macros add up to those amounts. Each time Joe enters a food or drink into his macro tracking app, it adds up the macros from each of those foods so he pays attention to this and chooses foods that will allow him to reach his goals of 276.5g carbs, 215g protein and 54.5g fats. Because Joe is fairly familiar with which foods have higher amounts of each macronutrient, he is able to select foods that he likes and by the end of the day have his macros add up to his goal amounts; success!

However, for someone just starting out with nutrition, it can be very difficult to know which foods to select to reach your goal macros when you don't know which foods are higher in a specific macronutrient. Even for those familiar with the nutrition in foods, it can be a bit difficult to decide what foods will allow you to reach your goals.

I found with many of my clients, there would come a time later in the day when they were close to their goal macros, but not quite there and they didn't know what foods they should have to get them there. The only way to go about it was basically trial and error, choosing a food, seeing what the macros were for it and deciding if it would help get closer to the goal amounts or not. This could be a tedious and time-consuming task to say the least.

I wanted to make this easier, so that even someone with no knowledge of the macros in foods could choose a food that would help them get closer to their macro goals with less effort and in less time. So I created a quick solution for this, a macro cheat sheet!

This cheat sheet gives you an easy to understand, quick visual of which foods are highest in each specific macronutrient. Some foods are highest in protein, some highest in carbs, some highest in fats, and some are high in more than one. With this cheat sheet you can see exactly where these foods land and choose a food to help you reach your macros more quickly and easily than ever before!

I have this cheat sheet attached right to my fridge with magnets so that if I find myself in need of more protein and fats, but not many carbs, I look at the list find Eggs in the overlapping section of protein and fats and voila! I can instantly see that Eggs will help me reach my protein and fat goals without putting me over on my carbs.

This has really made things easier for hitting macros and really helped speed up the process of choosing the proper foods. Also by having this visual display of which foods are higher in which macro, it allows people to more easily understand the nutrition in foods. In the end, this has turned out to be a helpful time-saver as well as a valuable educational tool in helping clients understand the macros in foods.

You can view the cheat sheet on the following page, and if you would like your own print out to stick on your fridge, visit: www.IIFYMbook.com/Macro-Cheat-Sheet to download your copy, absolutely free!

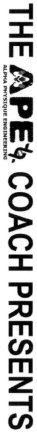

# THE APE COACH PRESENTS
### ALPHA PHYSIQUE ENGINEERING

## IIFYM Flexible Dieting Bodybuilding Guide

# MACRO CHEAT SHEET

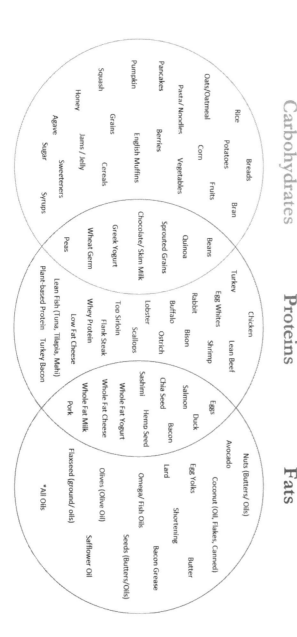

### Carbohydrates

Breads
Rice
Potatoes
Bran
Oats/Oatmeal
Corn
Fruits
Pasta / Noodles
Vegetables
Pancakes
Berries
English Muffins
Pumpkin
Grains
Cereals
Squash
Honey
Jams / Jelly
Agave
Sugar
Sweeteners
Syrups

Beans
Quinoa
Sprouted Grains
Chocolate/ Skim Milk
Greek Yogurt
Wheat Germ
Peas

### Proteins

Chicken
Turkey
Lean Beef
Egg Whites
Shrimp
Rabbit
Bison
Buffalo
Ostrich
Lobster
Scallops
Top Sirloin
Flank Steak
Whey Protein
Low Fat Cheese
Lean Fish (Tuna, Tilapia, Mahi)
Plant-based Protein   Turkey Bacon

Eggs
Salmon
Duck
Chia Seed
Bacon
Sashimi
Hemp Seed
Whole Fat Yogurt
Whole Fat Cheese
Whole Fat Milk
Pork

### Fats

Avocado
Nuts (Butters/ Oils)
Coconut (Oil, Flakes, Canned)
Lard
Egg Yolks
Shortening
Butter
Omega/ Fish Oils
Bacon Grease
Olives (Olive Oil)
Seeds (Butters/Oils)
Safflower Oil
Flaxseed (ground / oils)
*All Oils

81

*Chapter XIV*
# STEP FOUR –
# GET A FOOD SCALE

A lot of nutritional information is available on food packaging; however, a scale will ensure you accurately track what you eat. They are very inexpensive (normally costing between $20-$40) and can be found at most department stores (i.e. Walmart, Canadian Tire).

You can track your food and drinks simply by volume or general amounts (such as 1 medium apple or ½ Cup Oats); but measuring by volume or in general terms leaves a lot of room for error. One ½ Cup measuring cup when weighed may weigh 60g, while another "½ Cup" may weigh 80g.

There is just too much variability with volume measurements. Whereas weight is always the same. 100g of spinach always weighs 100g.

So if you want to get the best results, and you want to really make sure you are hitting your macros, the best thing to do is enter foods in weight and weigh your foods that you enter in your macro tracker with a food scale.

They are well worth the small investment for increasing how accurately you reach your macros and will be your second best friend!

*Chapter XV*
# STEP FIVE –
# MEASURE YOUR PROGRESS
# AND ADJUST

Now you're ready! You have all the tools and resources necessary to create your plan and achieve your ultimate dream body, fitness and health. But remember, without action, we only have a dream; so right now, today, I want you to start tracking your foods!

Enter in the app what you ate for breakfast, what you ate for lunch, and dinner, and any snacks or drinks you had throughout the day. This will take time, and it may be a bit challenging at first because it is something new. But this is the action that is going to take you one step closer to that dream vision of yours! And every time you enter your foods and use the app and track things, it becomes a little easier, you get a little better and a little quicker. And these consistent small action steps are what will produce the results you want to achieve in your health, fitness and physique to truly improve the quality of your life.

Every step forward builds momentum on the one before it and so by starting right now, you are creating a snowball effect to create and maintain your ultimate physique more rapidly than ever before.

You know everything you need to get you started on your new fitness and nutrition journey, but as we know, losing fat or building muscle isn't the hardest part, maintaining your results is.

The best way to ensure you are able to maintain your hard-earned results is to measure your progress along the way, track your weight, your body measurements, have your body composition tested and take photos to have physical evidence of your transformation.

As you lose or gain weight over time it is important to continually make adjustments to keep progressing and improving! Plus it's extremely motivating to have an account of your transformation journey. It allows you to really appreciate the process you put into attaining your goals.

Like many things in life, it's not always just about the end goal. This is a journey towards better health and fitness for life. This is a process to be enjoyed and celebrated as you reach each mini milestone along your path to your ultimate physique!

If you followed along and you apply each of the simple steps and utilize the tools and resources presented in this book, I know you will absolutely create greater results in your life than ever before.

Also, I love hearing all the dramatic, life changing transformations and accomplishments that individuals are able to accomplish from my programs and services. So if this book has helped you and you have a story you would like to share to inspire millions of others just like you, please submit your story, your transformation photos, your experience or your journey at www.IIFYMbook.com/Success-Stories.

And if you would like more individual attention, support, or accountability, please take the action right now and apply for my exclusive one-on-one online coaching program at: www.APEcoach.com/Coaching.

*Chapter XVI*
# BONUS –
# IIFYM FLEXIBLE DIETING
# BODYBUILDING RECIPES

By popular demand, after being requested by several clients, friends, family and the like to include some fantastic recipes in the book; I have decided to share with you some incredible IIFYM Flexible Dieting Bodybuilding Recipes as a bonus and thank you for buying the book!

The following are my Top Ten Favourite IIFYM Flexible Dieting Bodybuilding Recipes:

# GREEK YOGURT PROTEIN PANCAKES

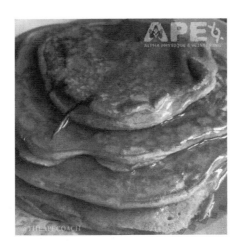

## INGREDIENTS:

| | |
|---|---|
| 1/3 Cup (90g) | **0% Plain Greek Yogurt** |
| 2 (65g) | **Egg Whites** |
| 1/8 Cup (20g) | **Flour** |
| 1/2 Scoop (16g) | **Vanilla Cake Whey Protein** |
| 1/2 tsp (2g) | **Baking Soda** |
| 1/2 tsp (2g) | **Vanilla Extract** |
| To Taste | **Cinnamon / Stevia** |

Combine all ingredients in a medium bowl, mix just until combined. Preheat pan over medium heat. Pour batter into centre of pan and cook for approx. 2mins or until top starts to bubble, flip and cook for an additional 1-2mins on the other side until golden brown and cooked through. Serve with low sugar syrup or your favourite pancake toppings and devour!

## MACROS PER SERVING (MAKES 3 SERVINGS):

| CALORIES | PROTEIN | CARBS | FAT |
|---|---|---|---|
| 66 | 10g | 5.2g | 0.2g |

# APPLE CINNAMON FRENCH TOAST

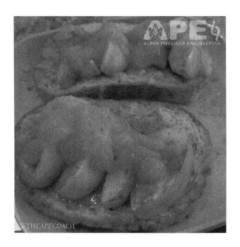

## INGREDIENTS:

| | |
|---|---|
| 2 Slices (60g) | **Light Rye Bread** |
| 2 (65g) | **Egg Whites** |
| 1/8 Cup (25g) | **Almond Milk** |
| 1/2 Scoop (16g) | **Vanilla Cake Whey Protein** |
| 1/2 tsp (2g) | **Vanilla Extract** |
| To Taste | **Cinnamon / Stevia** |
| 1/4 Cup (40g) | **Unsweetened Applesauce** |
| 1 (120g) | **Apple (Chopped)** |

Combine egg, milk, vanilla, cinnamon and stevia in a medium bowl, mix just until combined. Preheat pan over medium heat. Dip each side of rye bread in wet mix and place on pan and cook for approx. 2mins per side or until lightly browned. Top with chopped apple and applesauce, sprinkle extra cinnamon or stevia to taste and annihilate!

### MACROS PER SERVING (MAKES 2 SERVINGS):

| CALORIES | PROTEIN | CARBS | FAT |
|---|---|---|---|
| 165 | 12.9g | 27.4g | 0.6g |

# PROTEIN BANANA CHOCOLATE CHIP MUFFINS

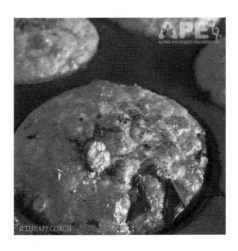

## INGREDIENTS:

| | | | |
|---|---|---|---|
| 3/4 Cup (90g) | **Large Flake Oats** | 1/4 Cup (64g) | **Unsweetened Applesauce** |
| Scoops (100g) | **Vanilla Cake Whey Protein** | 1 Tbsp (10g) | **Stevia** |
| 2 Med (220g) | **Banana (Mashed)** | 1/4 Cup (48g) | **Cocoa Powder** |
| | | 1/2 tsp (2g) | **Baking Soda** |
| 1/4 Cup (64g) | **0% Plain Greek Yogurt** | 1/2 tsp (2g) | **Baking Powder** |
| | | ¼ tsp (1g) | **Salt** |
| 1 Large (55g) | **Whole Egg** | 5 Tbsp (75g) | **Semisweet Chocolate Chips** |
| 1 Cup (186mL) | **Almond Milk** | | |

Combine all ingredients except chocolate chips in a food processor or blender. Preheat oven to 350ºF. Blend for 30sec-1min until well mixed. Pour batter into 12 serving muffin tin, evenly distribute chocolate chips on muffins. Bake at 350ºF for 18-20mins until toothpick inserted comes out clean. Let cool 10 minutes and decimate!

## MACROS PER SERVING (MAKES 12 SERVINGS):

| CALORIES | PROTEIN | CARBS | FAT |
|---|---|---|---|
| 115 | 9.1g | 14.7g | 3.4g |

# BODYBUILDING POPCORN CHICKEN

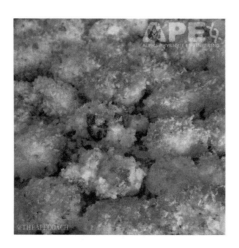

## INGREDIENTS:

| | |
|---|---|
| 2-3 (18oz) | **Boneless Skinless Chicken Breast** |
| 1 (55g) | **Whole Egg** |
| 2 XL (75g) | **Egg Whites** |
| 2 Tbsp (30mL) | **Original BBQ Sauce** |
| 1 Cup (120g) | **Bread Crumbs** |
| 1/2 tsp (2g) | **Garlic Powder** |
| 1/4 tsp (1g) | **Cayenne Pepper** |

Combine dry ingredients, except chicken in a bowl and combine wet ingredients in separate bowl. Cut chicken breast into 1 inch pieces. Dip chicken pieces in the wet mix and then coat in the dry mix to cover them. Place on a baking sheet sprayed with non-stick cooking spray. Bake at 450°F for 18-23mins and demolish!

## MACROS PER SERVING (MAKES 6 SERVINGS):

| CALORIES | PROTEIN | CARBS | FAT |
|---|---|---|---|
| 241 | 32.3g | 16.5g | 4.9g |

# BODYBUILDING GRILLED CHEESE

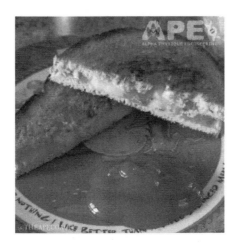

## INGREDIENTS:

2 Slices (60g) **Light Rye Bread**
2 oz. (60g) **Skim Milk (Allegro) Cheese**
2 Tbsp (30g) **Ketchup**

Heat a pan on medium heat. Spray with non-stick cooking spray. Cut cheese into thin strips and place between 2 slices of bread. Spray top and bottom of bread with cooking spray and place in middle of pan. Heat for a few minutes each side until golden brown and cheese is melted. Cut in half, serve with ketchup and obliterate!

## MACROS PER SERVING (MAKES 1 SERVING):

| CALORIES | PROTEIN | CARBS | FAT |
|----------|---------|-------|------|
| 289 | 28.5g | 41.5g | 2.1g |

# GARLIC PARM BROCCOLI PATTIES

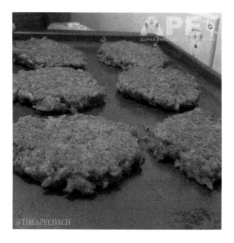

## INGREDIENTS:

| | |
|---|---|
| 2 Heads (350g) | **Broccoli (Florets)** |
| 1 (55g) | **Whole Egg** |
| 1/2 Cup (60g) | **Flour (Any)** |
| 1 tsp (5g) | **Garlic Clove (Minced)** |
| 1/4 Cup (60g) | **Parmesan Cheese (Grated)** |
| 1/8 Cup (30mL) | **Milk (Any)** |
| 1/2 tsp (2g) | **Salt** |
| 1/4 tsp (1g) | **Black Pepper (Ground)** |

Chop broccoli into florets, and steam until softened (5-10mins). Mix all other ingredients in a mixing bowl. Mash broccoli up with fork and combine with the rest of the ingredients. Mix until well combined. Heat pan on medium heat sprayed with cooking spray. Form the broccoli mix into patties and fry 3 patties at a time on pan for approx. 3 minutes each side until browned. Serve warm and destroy!

## MACROS PER SERVING (MAKES 7 SERVINGS):

| CALORIES | PROTEIN | CARBS | FAT |
|---|---|---|---|
| 73 | 4.2g | 10.6g | 1.8g |

# FAT-FREE BAKED SWEET POTATO FRIES

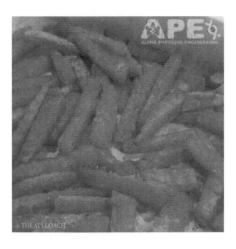

## INGREDIENTS:

| | |
|---|---|
| 2 (455g) | **Sweet Potatoes** |
| 1 tsp (5g) | **Corn Starch** |
| 1 tsp (5g) | **Sea Salt** |
| 1/2 tsp (2g) | **Black Pepper (Ground)** |
| 1/2 tsp (2g) | **Cinnamon** |
| 1/4 tsp (1g) | **Cayenne Pepper** |

Wash and peel sweet potatoes. Cut into thin ¼ inch fry-sized strips (I used a wavy cutter to make crinkle cut fries). Place fries in a mixing bowl, spray with non-stick cooking spray and add starch and spices. Toss in bowl until well coated. Add spices to taste. Spread evenly on a parchment paper lined baking sheet, with some space between fries and bake at 400°F for approx. 30mins flipping halfway until golden brown and crispy on the outside. Serve with a main dish or just gobble them on their own!

## MACROS PER SERVING (MAKES 4 SERVINGS):

| CALORIES | PROTEIN | CARBS | FAT |
|---|---|---|---|
| 102 | 2.4g | 23.8g | 0g |

# PROTEIN PUMPKIN PIE

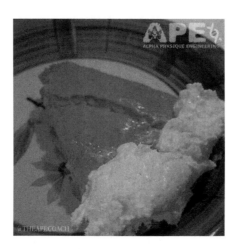

## INGREDIENTS:

| | |
|---|---|
| 1/2 Can (425g) | **Pumpkin Pure** |
| 2 Scoops (65g) | **Cinnamon Swirl Whey Protein** |
| 1 Cup (126g) | **Egg Whites** |
| 1/4 Cup (10g) | **Stevia** |
| 1/4 Cup (63mL) | **Almond Milk** |
| 1/4 Cup (63g) | **Fat Free Cream Cheese** |
| 1/2 tsp (2g) | **Vanilla Extract** |
| 1 ½ tsp (6g) | **Cinnamon** |
| 1/4 tsp (1g) each | **Ginger & Nutmeg** |
| 1/8 tsp (0.5g) | **Cloves** |

Combine all ingredients in a food processor or blender. Blend for approx. 1 minute until well blended. Pour into a 10inch pie dish sprayed with non-stick cooking spray. Bake at 350°F for 30mins then reduce temperature to 300°F and continue baking for approx. 15mins. Let cool slightly, top with fat free whipped cream or your favourite low cal toppings, cut into 8 slices and obliterate!

## MACROS PER SERVING (MAKES 8 SERVINGS):

| CALORIES | PROTEIN | CARBS | FAT |
|---|---|---|---|
| 80 | 9.8g | 7g | 0.8g |

# PROTEIN STRAWBERRY CHEESECAKE

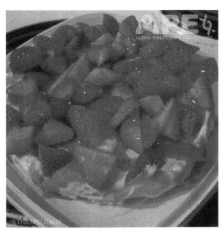

## INGREDIENTS:

**Cheesecake Mix:**

| | |
|---|---|
| 2 Scoops (70g) | **Vanilla or Strawberry Whey Protein** |
| 1 tsp (4g) | **Stevia** |
| 3/4 Cup (160g) | **Fat Free Cream Cheese** |
| 3/4 Cup (160g) | **0% Plain Greek Yogurt** |
| 1 Cup (126g) | **Egg Whites** |
| 4 tsp (20g) | **Unsweetened Applesauce** |
| 1 tsp (4g) | **Cinnamon** |
| 1/2 Cup (100g) | **Strawberries (Sliced)** |

**Icing:**

| | |
|---|---|
| 1/4 Cup (75g) | **Fat Free Cream Cheese** |
| 1/4 Cup (75g) | **0% Vanilla Greek Yogurt** |
| 1 tsp (4g) | **Stevia** |
| 1/2 tsp (2g) | **Vanilla Extract** |
| 1/4 Cup (25g) | **0 Cal Strawberry Syrup** |
| 1/2 Cup (100g) | **Strawberries (Sliced)** |

Combine all cake mix ingredients in a medium bowl, mix until well combined. Pour cake mix into 9" cake pan sprayed with non-stick cooking spray. Bake at 325°F for approx. 15mins, then reduce temperature to 180°F and continue baking for 35-40mins. Test with toothpick to check if done, it is okay if a little cake comes out on toothpick (you want the cheesecake moist still not dried out). Mix Icing ingredients in a bowl, spread on cake, add remaining strawberry slices and drizzle strawberry syrup. Cut into 8 slices and obliterate!

## MACROS PER SERVING (MAKES 8 SERVINGS):

| CALORIES | PROTEIN | CARBS | FAT |
|---|---|---|---|
| 119 | 15g | 8.5g | 2.1g |

# CHEESECAKE / PIE CRUST

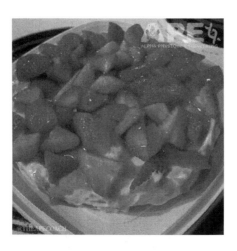

## INGREDIENTS:

| | |
|---|---|
| 1/2 Cup (60g) | **Flour** |
| 1/4 Cup (30g) | **Oat Flour (Ground Oats)** |
| 1/4 Cup (60g) | **Unsweetened Applesauce** |
| 1/2 tsp (2g) | **Stevia** |
| 1/2 tsp (2g) | **Cinnamon** |

Combine all ingredients in a medium bowl, mix until well combined. Press batter into thin layer on the bottom of cake pan or pie dish before adding the cake or pie mix. Bake according to cake or pie recipe. Cut into 8 servings and enjoy!

(Remember to add the macros for the crust to the cake or pie recipe to get accurate macros for your delicious dessert!)

## MACROS PER SERVING (MAKES 8 SERVINGS):

| CALORIES | PROTEIN | CARBS | FAT |
|----------|---------|-------|------|
| 43 | 1.4g | 9g | 0.3g |

# CLOSING WORDS

I don't care if you weigh 250lbs or 100lbs, because where you start is irrelevant, we all start somewhere. It's where you end up that really counts and the journey you take to get there.

Don't worry about where you're starting, focus on where you'll finish. We all begin at different ends of the spectrum, but in the end it's all about how we finish and what we accomplish, not where we began. Train and eat better today for a better tomorrow.

Do the things others won't do today, to do the things they can't do in the future. There are no shortcuts to any place worth going, and if something is worth doing at all, it is worth doing right. Building muscle or burning fat is no different.

Work your ass off, follow these principles closely, and I promise that your life will forever change for the better!

**Thanks for Reading!**

Tyler Johnston "The APE Coach"

www.APEcoach.com Presents:

# THANK YOU

**Mom** – For raising me and teaching me the morals and values that shape my life today. For taking me to all those practices and allowing me to participate in so many sports growing up. For always loving and supporting me in everything I have done and being there to cheer me on every step of the way. For buying groceries and understanding my crazy contest preparation processes more and more. I would not be where I am or who I am without you.

**Tabitha** – For always being there to support me and encourage me. You've believed in me, with all of my crazy ideas and dreams even when I wasn't sure if, or how they would work out. You put up with this wild lifestyle of fitness, nutrition and entrepreneurship and the stress and emotions in competing. Your unconditional love and caring has made me a better man. I always know I can count on you if my confidence ever begins to waiver. You are my rock and I love you with all of my heart.

**Rob** – For showing me this world of fitness and pushing me to constantly be better since we were little kids. You introduced me to fitness and showed me how to build strength with our push up, chin up and sit up contests before I ever knew what fitness even was. Without you showing me the way and getting me started I may never have ended up achieving all I have today or discovered my insatiable passion for fitness and health. Thanks for being an awesome big brother.

**Scott Mclelland** – For working with me and showing me a whole new side of the world of fitness. You are much more than my coach, I consider you a dear friend and know I can trust you to always push me to be my absolute best. Without you I never would have gotten to the level I have with my fitness and health, and for that I am forever grateful!

**Dad** – For introducing me to Anthony Robbins and the world of personal development. For showing me it is possible to create your own life and future, to be your own boss and determine your own worth. Without the personal development and leadership opportunities I've had the privilege to take part in, I would not have had the belief or skills to make any of this possible.

**Luis Angel** – For believing in me and my work. For inspiring me to reach for more, to raise my standards and create something beyond what I would have ever imagined with this project. This book would not be near what it now is without you.

**Other Thank You's Go To** – Krystalyn, Kieran, my grandparents, my entire family, Sadik, Arnie, Sly, Tony, all of my coaches and role models and idols who have pushed me in the past. I would also like to thank the Global Youth Leadership Summit and everyone else who has supported me, inspired me and motivated me to be and do more with my life and helped me along the way!

# ABOUT THE AUTHOR

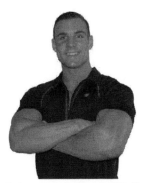

*Tyler Johnston "The APE Coach"*

- **Founder** and Head Training/ Fitness Nutrition Coach at Alpha Physique Engineering
- **Certified** Personal Training Specialist
- **Certified** Fitness Nutrition Coach
- **Won 1st** Men's Physique Medium at Guelph Mo-Muscle Classic
- **Won 1st** Mr. CHIN Fitness Model 2014
- **Nationally Qualified** CBBF Natural Men's Physique Competitor
- **Holds Degrees** in Psychology and Business Administration from Wilfrid Laurier University
- **Amazon International Best-selling Author** and Creator of "The APE Coach Presents" Series: IIFYM Flexible Dieting Bodybuilding Guide.

www.APEcoach.com Presents:

# LEARN MORE / CONTACT

Learn more about Tyler Johnston's "The APE Coach Presents" programs and other fitness and nutrition material for Bodybuilders, Physique Athletes, Fitness Beginners, Professionals, and everyone else, by going to: **www.APEcoach.com**

## SOCIAL
**FB:** www.Facebook.com/theAPEcoach
**YT:** www.Youtube.com/APEcoach
**IG:** @THEAPECOACH
**Twitter:** @THEAPECOACH
**Email:** info@APEcoach.com

15696884R00058

Printed in Great Britain
by Amazon